The Digestion Fix

Why Your Body Can't Handle Food and How to Restore It

First Edition: March 2026
ISBN: 978-1-966035-02-2
Published by Elite Nutrition Research
EliteNutritionResearch.com

Table of Contents

INTRODUCTION

DIGESTION IS NOT ABOUT FOOD

Digestion is commonly framed as a question of food choice, as if outcomes are determined primarily by what enters the mouth. This framing collapses a complex system into a single variable and ignores the machinery that actually processes that input. The body does not respond to food in isolation. It responds to food through a sequence of coordinated events that determine whether that food is broken down, absorbed, and integrated, or whether it lingers, ferments, and becomes a source of stress. The same meal can produce radically different outcomes depending on the state and capacity of the system receiving it. What appears as food sensitivity, intolerance, or poor dietary compatibility is often a reflection of incomplete processing rather than an inherent problem with the food itself.

The digestive system operates as a chain of transformations. Food must be mechanically reduced, chemically unfolded, enzymatically cleaved, emulsified into transportable structures, and then moved across membranes into circulation. Each stage depends on the precision of the stage before it. If stomach acid fails to reach sufficient strength, proteins remain partially folded and resistant to enzymatic access. If proteins are not properly unfolded, downstream enzymes encounter substrates that are structurally intact and difficult to cleave. If enzymatic breakdown is incomplete, the small intestine receives larger fragments that cannot be efficiently absorbed. These fragments alter osmotic gradients, disrupt motility, and create conditions that favor fermentation. The system does not fail at a single point and stop. It continues forward in a degraded state, carrying inefficiencies into every subsequent step.

This is why symptoms rarely localize cleanly to one organ. Bloating, reflux, irregular bowel movements, and food reactions are not isolated malfunctions but expressions of a system that has lost sequence integrity. When early steps weaken, later steps attempt to compensate. The intestine may slow transit to allow more time for breakdown, or accelerate transit to move problematic material through more quickly. Microbial populations shift in response to the substrates that arrive, expanding where undigested material accumulates. The immune system becomes more active as larger, partially processed molecules interact with the intestinal barrier. What presents as a collection of unrelated symptoms is often the predictable output of a system that is no longer operating in the correct order.

The focus on food alone creates a misleading feedback loop. When digestion is compromised, certain foods consistently produce discomfort. Those foods are then removed, which can reduce symptoms in the short term but does not restore the underlying capacity of the system. Over time, the range of tolerable foods narrows because the system itself has not been repaired. The threshold for reaction drops, and increasingly simple inputs begin to cause the same problems. This progression is often interpreted as the body becoming more sensitive, but the underlying issue is that the system has lost the ability to fully process even basic substrates.

A more accurate model begins with capacity rather than selection. The digestive system must be able to generate sufficient acid, enzymes, and bile, coordinate timing between organs, maintain proper motility, and preserve the integrity of the intestinal barrier. When these elements are functioning together, a wide range of foods can be processed with minimal disturbance. When they are not, even carefully selected diets produce inconsistent results. The goal is not to find the perfect set of foods that avoid symptoms, but to restore the sequence that allows food to be converted into usable material.

This reframing changes how digestion is approached. Instead of asking which foods are safe or unsafe, the question becomes whether the system can perform the transformations required to handle them. Instead of treating symptoms as isolated problems, they are understood as outputs that reflect where the sequence is breaking down. Restoration then follows the structure of the system itself, rebuilding each step so that inputs can move through without creating disruption. When the sequence is restored, digestion becomes predictable again, and food returns to its proper role as a source of structure rather than a trigger for instability.

Digestion is not governed by the identity of food as much as it is governed by the condition of the system receiving it. Food is an input. Digestion is the process that determines what that input becomes. When the system is intact, inputs are transformed into amino acids, fatty acids, minerals, and signaling molecules that can be absorbed, transported, and built into cellular structure. When the system is degraded, those same inputs remain partially processed, mechanically altered but chemically incomplete, and they move forward as unstable material that disrupts downstream function. The difference between tolerance and reaction is not primarily located in the food itself. It is located in the sequence of transformations that the body is able to execute.

This sequence begins before food is swallowed and continues through multiple coordinated phases that depend on timing, signaling, and fluid dynamics. Sensory input prepares the system, gastric acid unfolds protein structure, enzymes cleave macromolecules into smaller units, bile organizes lipids into transportable forms, and the intestinal lining regulates what enters circulation. Each phase is constrained by the performance of the phase before it. If gastric output is insufficient, the chemical structure of incoming material remains resistant to enzymatic action. If enzymatic breakdown is incomplete, the intestine is forced to handle substrates that exceed its absorptive capacity. What follows is not a clean failure but a shift into compensation. Transit patterns change, microbial activity increases, and immune exposure rises as larger fragments interact with the barrier.

Focusing on food selection alone ignores this structure. It assumes that removing inputs will solve problems that are actually being generated by processing inefficiency. This approach can reduce symptoms by lowering the demand placed on the system, but it does not rebuild the system itself. Over time, the range of tolerable inputs narrows because the underlying capacity continues to decline. Foods that were once manageable begin to produce the same outcomes because the system no longer has the strength to complete the required transformations. What appears as increasing sensitivity is a reduction in processing capability.

A coordinated system behaves differently. It does not depend on narrow inputs to maintain stability. It maintains stability by executing each stage of digestion with sufficient precision that inputs are consistently converted into usable material. When acid production reaches effective levels, proteins lose their structural resistance and become accessible to enzymes. When enzymes are released in the correct quantities and timing, macromolecules are reduced to absorbable units. When bile flow is sufficient, fats are emulsified into structures that can be transported across membranes. The system becomes less reactive because it is no longer carrying incomplete material forward.

Understanding digestion as a coordinated system shifts the objective away from managing inputs and toward restoring function. Food becomes secondary to the architecture that processes it. The focus moves to rebuilding sequence integrity, increasing output where it has declined, and restoring the timing between stages so that each step prepares the next. As this structure is re-established, the system regains the ability to handle a broader range of inputs without instability. The outcome is not dependent on finding the right foods but on restoring the conditions under which food can be fully processed.

Sequence Failure vs Food Blame

When digestion breaks down, the failure rarely occurs at the level of food itself. It occurs in the sequence that processes that food. The system depends on ordered transformations, where each step prepares the substrate for the next. When that order is disrupted, the output changes even if the input remains the same. A meal that would normally be reduced into absorbable components instead moves forward in a partially processed state. Proteins remain structurally intact, fats are insufficiently emulsified, and carbohydrates persist in forms that alter fluid balance within the intestine. The system continues to move this material downstream, but it does so under degraded conditions that amplify instability at every stage.

Blame is often assigned to the food because the symptoms appear after eating, but the timing obscures the real mechanism. Food exposes the system's current capacity. If stomach acid is insufficient, protein does not fully unfold. If protein structure remains intact, enzymes encounter resistance at the molecular level and cleavage becomes inefficient. If enzymatic breakdown is incomplete, larger fragments enter the intestine where they disrupt osmotic gradients, interfere with coordinated motility, and increase microbial activity. Gas production, pressure, irregular transit, and immune activation follow. These outcomes are attributed to the food that initiated the sequence, but the cause is the system's inability to complete the transformations required to process it.

This misattribution creates a reinforcing loop. A specific food produces discomfort and is removed, which reduces symptoms by lowering the processing demand placed on the system. The underlying inefficiency remains unchanged. Over time, other foods begin to produce similar effects because the system's capacity continues to decline. The range of tolerable inputs narrows, and the threshold for disruption becomes lower. What appears to be increasing sensitivity is a progressive loss of processing capability driven by unresolved sequence failure.

A sequence-based view explains why symptoms cluster and shift over time. The same upstream weakness can produce different downstream outputs depending on how the system compensates. If incoming material is poorly prepared in the stomach, the intestine may slow transit to allow additional breakdown, increasing retention and fermentation. In other cases, transit accelerates to move unstable material through more quickly, reducing absorption and increasing variability in bowel patterns. These are not separate conditions. They are different expressions of the same disruption in sequence integrity.

Restoring digestion requires rebuilding the order of operations rather than narrowing inputs. Each stage must regain sufficient output and timing so that material is fully transformed before it advances. Acid must alter protein structure to expose cleavage sites, enzymes must reduce macromolecules into absorbable units, bile must organize lipids into transportable forms, and the intestinal barrier must transfer these materials into circulation without excessive exposure to incomplete fragments. As sequence integrity returns, the system no longer carries forward unstable material, and foods that once triggered symptoms can be processed without disruption because the underlying machinery is functioning again.

Symptom Clustering as System Breakdown

Digestive symptoms rarely appear in isolation because the system itself is not isolated. It operates as a continuous chain of transformations, and when one segment loses precision, the effects propagate forward and alter the behavior of multiple downstream processes. What shows up as bloating, reflux, irregular bowel movements, fatigue, or skin irritation is not a collection of unrelated problems. It is a clustered output generated by a system that is no longer maintaining sequence integrity. Each symptom reflects a point where material is being handled under suboptimal conditions, and those conditions tend to overlap because the same upstream failure feeds multiple downstream disruptions.

When gastric processing is incomplete, the material entering the small intestine carries structural resistance. Proteins remain partially folded, fats remain poorly organized, and carbohydrates may not be fully reduced into simpler forms. This changes the physical and chemical environment of the intestine. Larger fragments alter osmotic gradients and draw fluid into the lumen. Motility becomes less coordinated as the system attempts to either slow down to allow more time for breakdown or speed up to clear material that is not being processed effectively. At the same time, microbial populations expand in response to the increased availability of fermentable substrates. Gas production rises, pressure builds, and the intestinal wall is exposed to compounds that would not normally be present in that concentration.

These changes do not remain confined to the gut. The intestinal barrier is forced to manage a higher load of partially processed material, increasing the likelihood that larger fragments interact with immune tissue. Immune activation follows, not as a primary dysfunction, but as a response to exposure that should have been prevented earlier in the sequence. Signaling molecules released during this process influence systemic physiology. Energy levels shift as nutrient extraction becomes inconsistent. The nervous system receives altered input from the gut, which can affect focus, mood, and stress responses. What appears as a wide range of unrelated symptoms is the system expressing the consequences of incomplete transformation at multiple levels.

Symptom clustering becomes more pronounced as the system adapts to its own inefficiency. If transit slows to compensate for poor breakdown, retention increases and fermentation becomes more dominant. If transit accelerates, absorption becomes inconsistent and the body experiences fluctuations in available nutrients. These opposing patterns can occur in the same individual over time because the system is not stable. It is reacting dynamically to the state of incoming material. This variability is often interpreted as multiple overlapping conditions, but it is more accurately understood as a single system producing different outputs depending on how it is compensating at that moment.

Viewing symptoms as a cluster rather than as isolated events changes how the problem is approached. Instead of treating each symptom independently, the focus shifts to the sequence that generates them.

Restoring upstream processing reduces the load placed on downstream systems, which in turn reduces the need for compensation. As acid production, enzymatic activity, and bile flow return to effective levels, the material entering the intestine becomes more uniform and easier to handle. Motility stabilizes because the system is no longer forced to adjust for poorly processed substrates. Microbial activity normalizes as excess fermentable material decreases. Immune exposure is reduced because fewer incomplete fragments reach the barrier. The cluster of symptoms resolves not through targeted suppression, but through the restoration of the system that produced them.

Food Intolerance as a Capacity Problem

Food intolerance is typically interpreted as a property of the food itself, as if certain inputs are inherently incompatible with the body. This interpretation ignores the role of processing capacity. Digestion is not a passive reaction to food. It is an active sequence that requires sufficient output at each stage to transform incoming material into absorbable components. When that output is reduced, the system loses the ability to complete those transformations, and the same food that was once handled without issue begins to produce symptoms. The intolerance is not embedded in the food. It emerges from the system's inability to process it.

Capacity is determined by multiple coordinated functions. The stomach must generate enough acid to alter protein structure and initiate breakdown. The pancreas must release enzymes in sufficient quantity and timing to reduce macromolecules into smaller units. The liver and gallbladder must supply bile to organize fats into emulsified structures that can be transported across the intestinal lining. The intestine itself must maintain a surface that can absorb these materials efficiently without allowing larger, incomplete fragments to pass through. When any part of this system underperforms, the burden shifts forward, and the material entering the next stage is more difficult to handle.

As capacity declines, the threshold for disruption lowers. Foods that require more extensive processing become problematic first because they place a higher demand on the system. Proteins that depend on strong acid for unfolding, fats that require coordinated bile release for emulsification, and complex carbohydrates that rely on enzymatic precision begin to produce inconsistent outcomes. When these foods are removed, symptoms often improve because the system is no longer being pushed beyond its limits. This creates the impression that the foods themselves were the problem, when in reality the system lacked the capacity to process them at that time.

Over time, if capacity is not restored, the range of tolerable foods continues to narrow. Simpler inputs begin to produce the same effects because even minimal processing demands exceed what the system can deliver. The body appears increasingly sensitive, but the underlying change is a progressive reduction in functional output. The system is operating closer to its limit with each input, and small variations in timing, stress, or meal composition can push it into instability. This is why food reactions often seem unpredictable. The variability reflects fluctuations in system capacity rather than inherent unpredictability in the foods themselves.

Restoring tolerance requires rebuilding capacity across the entire sequence. Acid production must reach levels that consistently alter protein structure. Enzymatic output must be sufficient to complete breakdown before material advances. Bile flow must be coordinated so that fats are properly emulsified and absorbed. The intestinal barrier must regain the ability to transfer nutrients while limiting exposure to incomplete fragments. As these functions recover, the system can handle progressively more complex inputs without exceeding its limits. Foods that once triggered symptoms can be reintroduced not because they have changed, but because the system processing them has regained the ability to complete the required transformations.

Core Thesis: Digestion Fails and Heals in Sequence

Digestion operates as an ordered chain of transformations, and the direction of change within that chain determines whether the system moves toward stability or dysfunction. Failure does not occur randomly. It follows the structure of the system itself. When an early step weakens, every downstream step is forced to operate on material that has not been properly prepared. The system continues to function, but it does so under constraint, carrying forward partially processed inputs that alter the behavior of each subsequent stage. This is why digestive issues tend to expand rather than remain contained. A disruption at the beginning of the sequence does not stay localized. It propagates.

The stomach represents the first major transformation point where structure is actively changed. Acid exposure unfolds protein and sets the conditions for enzymatic access. When this step is incomplete, the material entering the small intestine retains structural resistance. Enzymes encounter substrates that are more difficult to cleave, which reduces the efficiency of breakdown. Larger fragments persist, and the intestine must process material that exceeds its optimal operating range. This shifts the internal environment. Motility adjusts, fluid balance changes, and microbial activity increases in response to the altered substrate profile. The system adapts, but the adaptation introduces new inefficiencies that further distance it from its original operating state.

Downstream systems then begin to compensate for upstream failure. Bile release may become inconsistent because signaling from the stomach and upper intestine is altered. Fat emulsification becomes less effective, which interferes with absorption and changes the composition of material moving through the gut. The intestinal barrier is exposed to a higher load of incomplete fragments, increasing the likelihood of immune interaction. Energy extraction becomes less predictable because nutrients are not being fully reduced and absorbed. Each layer of compensation adds complexity, but none of it resolves the original problem. The system is attempting to manage the consequences of incomplete transformation rather than restoring the conditions required for proper transformation.

Healing follows the same structure in reverse. Restoration does not begin with the symptoms that appear at the end of the sequence. It begins with the steps that shape everything downstream. When gastric output is restored, proteins lose their structural resistance and become accessible to enzymes. When enzymatic breakdown improves, the intestine receives material that is closer to its absorbable form, reducing the need for compensatory adjustments. When bile flow becomes consistent, fats are organized into structures that can be transported efficiently, stabilizing both absorption and signaling. Each restored step reduces the burden on the next, allowing the system to return toward coordinated function.

This sequential model explains why isolated interventions often produce limited or temporary results. Supporting a downstream process without correcting upstream preparation leaves the system dependent on compensation. Improvements may occur, but they remain constrained by the unresolved inefficiency earlier in the chain. In contrast, restoring the sequence rebuilds the system's internal logic. Each stage begins to prepare the next in a way that reduces friction and increases predictability. Digestion becomes less reactive because inputs are no longer entering each phase in a compromised state.

The central principle is simple but often overlooked. The system can only perform as well as its earliest effective step. When that step fails, the entire chain adjusts around it. When that step is restored, the entire chain begins to reorganize toward normal function. Digestion does not fail all at once, and it does not heal all at once. It moves in sequence, and understanding that structure determines whether the system continues to fragment or begins to recover.

PART I

DIGESTION STARTS IN THE BRAIN

Chapter 1

The Digestive State

Digestion begins as a state, not as a reaction to food. Before any mechanical breakdown or chemical transformation occurs, the body must enter a mode that permits those processes to operate. This state is governed by the nervous system, specifically by the balance between parasympathetic and sympathetic activity. When parasympathetic signaling is dominant, the body allocates resources toward secretion, motility, and coordinated digestive output. Blood flow is directed toward the gastrointestinal tract, glands increase production of digestive fluids, and the sequence of events required for processing food is allowed to initiate. When sympathetic signaling dominates, those same processes are suppressed. Blood flow is redirected toward skeletal muscle, secretion is reduced, and motility becomes less coordinated. The system does not partially engage digestion under these conditions. It restricts it.

This state acts as a gatekeeper. Food entering the system does not automatically trigger full digestive function. The nervous system determines whether the system will operate at sufficient capacity to process that input. If the body is in a constrained state, the early stages of digestion are already compromised before food reaches the stomach. Salivary output may be reduced, sensory signaling is diminished, and the anticipatory phase that prepares the stomach and pancreas is weakened. By the time food arrives in the stomach, the system is already operating below its required output, and the sequence begins with a deficit.

Gastric function is particularly sensitive to this state. Acid production is not constant. It is modulated by neural input that reflects the body's readiness to digest. When parasympathetic tone is present, acid secretion increases to levels that can alter protein structure effectively. When sympathetic tone dominates, acid output is reduced. Proteins enter the stomach but are not exposed to sufficient acidity to unfold completely. This alters the entire downstream process. Enzymes that depend on unfolded substrates encounter resistance, and the material that moves into the small intestine carries structural integrity that should have been removed. The system is forced to compensate for a failure that occurred before digestion fully began.

Motility follows the same pattern. Coordinated movement of food through the digestive tract depends on rhythmic signaling that is supported by the parasympathetic system. When this signaling is disrupted, movement becomes irregular. Food may remain in the stomach longer than intended, increasing the opportunity for fermentation, or it may pass too quickly into the intestine without adequate preparation. In the small intestine, segmentation and peristalsis lose precision, which affects both breakdown and absorption. The system continues to move material forward, but it does so without the timing required to maintain efficiency.

This state-dependent behavior explains why digestion can vary significantly even when food intake remains consistent. A meal consumed in a calm, regulated state may be processed with minimal disturbance, while the same meal consumed under stress produces bloating, discomfort, or irregularity. The difference is not in the food. It is in the system's ability to enter a state that supports the sequence of digestion. Without that state, the system begins from a position of reduced capacity and carries that reduction through every subsequent step.

Chronic suppression of the digestive state leads to structural changes in how the system operates. When the body repeatedly processes food under constrained conditions, it adapts to that constraint. Secretory output remains low, motility patterns become inconsistent, and the coordination between organs weakens. The system begins to normalize dysfunction. What started as a temporary reduction in capacity becomes a persistent operating mode. Over time, this reduces tolerance to a wider range of foods because the system is no longer capable of executing the sequence at full capacity.

Restoring digestion requires restoring the state that permits it. This does not begin with food selection or supplementation. It begins with re-establishing the conditions under which the system is allowed to function. When parasympathetic signaling is restored, secretory output increases, motility becomes more coordinated, and the sequence can begin to operate as designed. Each step regains the ability to prepare the next, and the system moves away from compensation and back toward coordinated processing. The digestive state is not an accessory to digestion. It is the condition that determines whether digestion can occur at all.

Nervous System Control of Digestion

Digestion is directed by the nervous system before it is carried out by organs. The stomach, pancreas, liver, and intestine do not decide independently when to secrete or how strongly to contract. Their activity is driven by neural input that sets the level of output across the entire system. This control is primarily organized through the balance between parasympathetic and sympathetic signaling, with the enteric nervous system acting as a local network that executes instructions and adjusts behavior in real time. When parasympathetic tone is sufficient, secretion increases, motility becomes coordinated, and blood flow is directed toward the gastrointestinal tract. When sympathetic tone dominates, those same processes are reduced or suppressed, and the system shifts away from digestion toward immediate survival priorities.

The vagus nerve provides the main parasympathetic pathway that links the brain to the digestive organs. Its activity determines how strongly the stomach secretes acid, how effectively the pancreas releases enzymes, and how consistently the gallbladder contracts to deliver bile. This is not a subtle modulation. Changes in vagal output directly alter the volume and timing of digestive secretions. When vagal signaling is strong, gastric acid reaches levels that unfold protein structure, enzymes are released in synchrony with incoming material, and bile enters the intestine at the moment it is needed for fat emulsification. When vagal signaling is weak, each of these outputs is reduced. The system continues to function, but it does so below the threshold required for complete processing.

The enteric nervous system operates within the walls of the gastrointestinal tract and coordinates local activity, but it does not override the global state set by the central nervous system. It organizes peristalsis, segmentation, and local reflexes that move and mix material, but its behavior is constrained by the level of input it receives. If upstream signaling reduces secretion, the enteric network must work with material that is less prepared and more difficult to process. Motility patterns adjust in response to this altered substrate. Movement may slow to allow more time for breakdown, or accelerate to clear material that is not being handled efficiently. These adjustments are compensatory. They do not correct the underlying issue of reduced input from the central control system.

Blood flow is also regulated through neural control, and this directly affects digestive capacity. Under parasympathetic dominance, circulation is directed toward the stomach and intestines, supporting secretion, absorption, and tissue maintenance. Under sympathetic dominance, blood is diverted toward skeletal muscle and away from the digestive tract. This reduces the resources available for secretion and limits the ability of the intestinal lining to absorb nutrients efficiently. Even if enzymes and bile are present, reduced perfusion constrains how effectively the system can use them. The physical environment required for digestion is altered at the level of circulation.

This control system explains why digestion can change rapidly without any alteration in diet. A shift in nervous system state can increase or decrease acid production, enzyme release, bile flow, and motility within a short time frame. The same meal can be processed efficiently or poorly depending on whether the system is receiving signals that permit full operation. When neural control is consistently biased toward suppression, the system adapts to a lower baseline of activity. Secretory glands reduce output, motility patterns become irregular, and coordination between organs weakens. The system is still active, but it operates with reduced precision and lower capacity.

Restoring digestion requires restoring the signaling that drives it. The organs involved in digestion respond to instruction. When parasympathetic signaling increases, secretion rises, timing improves, and the sequence of digestion begins to reassemble into a coordinated process. The enteric nervous system can then operate on material that has been properly prepared, and motility stabilizes because it no longer needs to compensate for upstream inefficiency. The control layer determines the performance of the entire system, and without correcting it, downstream interventions remain limited by the signals that continue to restrict output.

Parasympathetic Dominance and Digestive Permission

Digestion requires permission at the level of the nervous system before it can proceed at full capacity. This permission is granted through parasympathetic dominance, which shifts the body into a mode where resources are allocated toward processing, absorption, and internal maintenance. Without this shift, the digestive system does not fully engage. It operates in a restricted state, producing lower levels of acid, enzymes, and bile, while motility becomes less coordinated and blood flow is directed away from the gastrointestinal tract. The system is active, but it is not operating with the output required to complete the sequence of digestion.

Parasympathetic signaling initiates the preparatory phase that allows digestion to begin before food is even swallowed. Sensory input from sight, smell, and taste activates neural pathways that increase salivary secretion and prime the stomach for acid production. This early signaling sets the baseline for everything that follows. When parasympathetic tone is strong, gastric glands are activated in advance, and the stomach is ready to alter protein structure as soon as food arrives. When this signaling is weak or absent, the system starts behind, and the stomach must attempt to generate sufficient output after the fact. This delay reduces the effectiveness of the initial transformation and alters the quality of material that moves forward.

Gastric acid production is directly tied to this state. Under parasympathetic dominance, acid secretion reaches levels that denature proteins and create an environment where enzymatic activity can proceed efficiently. The pH of the stomach is not a static value but a controlled condition that depends on neural input. When sympathetic signaling overrides parasympathetic activity, acid production is reduced. Proteins remain partially folded, and the stomach becomes a holding chamber rather than an active processing site. The material that exits the stomach carries structural resistance into the small intestine, increasing the burden on downstream systems.

Pancreatic enzyme release and bile flow follow the same pattern. Parasympathetic input coordinates the timing and quantity of these secretions so that they match the arrival of partially processed material from the stomach. Enzymes are delivered in concentrations that can complete the breakdown of macromolecules, and bile is released in a way that allows fats to be emulsified into absorbable structures. When parasympathetic signaling is reduced, these outputs become inconsistent. Enzymes may be released in insufficient amounts or at the wrong time, and bile flow may not align with the presence of dietary fats. The system loses synchronization, and each stage operates with reduced efficiency.

Motility is also governed by this permission state. Under parasympathetic dominance, the digestive tract moves material in coordinated patterns that allow for thorough mixing and controlled progression. The stomach empties at a rate that reflects the level of processing achieved, and the small intestine segments and propels material in a way that maximizes contact with digestive surfaces. When this state is suppressed, motility becomes irregular. Food may remain in the stomach longer than necessary or pass too quickly into the intestine without adequate preparation. In the small intestine, segmentation loses precision, reducing the effectiveness of both breakdown and absorption.

Digestive permission is not an abstract concept. It is a measurable shift in output across the entire system. When parasympathetic signaling is present, secretion increases, timing improves, and the physical environment required for digestion is established. When it is absent, the system operates under constraint, and every stage begins with a deficit that carries forward. The difference between efficient digestion and chronic instability often begins at this level. Without permission, the system cannot perform the transformations required to convert food into usable material. With it, the sequence can proceed with the precision needed to maintain stability.

Stress as a Suppressor of Digestive Output

Stress shifts the body into a state where digestion is deprioritized at the level of control, not at the level of food. Sympathetic activation alters the allocation of resources, directing blood flow toward skeletal muscle and away from the gastrointestinal tract, reducing secretory output, and disrupting the timing that coordinates each stage of digestion. The system does not shut off completely, but it operates below the threshold required to complete the sequence. Acid production drops, enzyme release becomes inconsistent, bile flow loses synchronization, and motility patterns become irregular. Material continues to move through the system, but it is processed under constrained conditions that favor incomplete transformation.

Gastric function is one of the first areas affected. Acid secretion depends on neural input that reflects whether the body is in a state that permits digestion. Under stress, that input is reduced, and the stomach produces less acid. Proteins enter but are not fully denatured, which limits enzymatic access later in the process. The stomach retains food longer as it attempts to compensate for reduced chemical breakdown, increasing the likelihood of fermentation and pressure buildup. In some cases, the system accelerates emptying to move inadequately processed material into the intestine, trading preparation for speed. Both patterns originate from the same constraint. The stomach is operating without sufficient output.

Pancreatic and biliary responses are also altered. Enzyme secretion depends on coordinated signaling between the stomach, intestine, and nervous system. When stress disrupts that signaling, enzymes may be released in lower quantities or at the wrong time relative to incoming material. Bile release becomes less predictable, which affects fat emulsification and the formation of structures required for absorption. Fats pass through the system in larger, less organized forms, increasing the burden on the intestine and altering the composition of material that reaches the colon. The downstream environment shifts as a result, not because of the food itself, but because of how it was processed.

Motility changes under stress in ways that reflect the system's attempt to manage incomplete processing. Peristalsis and segmentation lose coordination, leading to either slowed transit with increased retention or accelerated transit with reduced absorption. These opposing patterns can occur within the same individual depending on how the system responds at a given moment. When transit slows, fermentation becomes more prominent as microbial populations act on substrates that were not fully broken down. When transit accelerates, nutrients pass through before they can be absorbed, leading to variability in energy availability and nutrient status. The system adapts to constraint, but the adaptation introduces new inefficiencies.

Circulatory changes reinforce these effects. Reduced blood flow to the digestive organs limits both secretion and absorption. Even when enzymes and bile are present, the tissues responsible for processing and transport operate with fewer resources. The intestinal lining has less capacity to move nutrients across membranes and maintain barrier integrity. Larger fragments are more likely to interact with immune tissue, increasing the probability of inflammatory signaling. These changes are not isolated. They are coordinated responses to a state that deprioritizes digestion at multiple levels simultaneously.

Chronic stress extends these patterns into a stable operating mode. When the system repeatedly processes food under constrained conditions, it adapts by lowering baseline output. Secretory capacity declines, timing between organs becomes less precise, and the coordination required for efficient digestion weakens. Symptoms become more consistent because the system is consistently operating below capacity. Food appears to be the trigger, but the underlying condition is a control state that limits the system's ability to perform the necessary transformations.

Restoring digestive function requires reversing this suppression at the level of control. As sympathetic dominance decreases and parasympathetic signaling increases, secretion rises, timing improves, and blood flow returns to the gastrointestinal tract. The stomach regains the ability to generate sufficient acid, the pancreas and liver restore coordinated output, and motility stabilizes because material is being properly prepared at each stage. The system no longer needs to compensate for incomplete processing. Digestion becomes more predictable because the conditions required for full transformation are present again.

State-Dependent Digestion Variability

Digestion does not produce consistent outcomes from identical inputs because the system that processes those inputs is not constant. The digestive tract operates according to the state imposed by the nervous system, and that state can shift from one meal to the next without any change in diet. Acid output, enzyme release, bile flow, motility, and blood distribution all respond to this control layer. When the state supports digestion, these processes align in timing and magnitude. When the state constrains digestion, each process operates below capacity or out of sequence. The variability observed in symptoms is a direct reflection of these shifting conditions rather than an inherent unpredictability in the food itself.

Gastric performance illustrates this clearly. In a state that permits digestion, the stomach generates acid at levels that unfold protein structure early in the process. The material that exits the stomach is chemically altered and ready for enzymatic reduction. In a constrained state, acid output is lower, and proteins remain partially intact. The same meal enters the small intestine in two different forms depending on the state under which it was processed. Enzymes encounter either an accessible substrate or one that resists cleavage, and the efficiency of breakdown diverges immediately. The difference is established before the intestine has an opportunity to act.

Pancreatic and biliary responses amplify this divergence. When signaling is intact, enzyme release is synchronized with the arrival of partially processed material, and bile is delivered in a pattern that supports fat emulsification. Lipids are organized into structures that can be transported across the intestinal lining, and the system proceeds with predictable absorption. When the state is constrained, enzyme output may be delayed or insufficient, and bile release may not match the presence of dietary fat. The same fat intake can be efficiently emulsified in one state and poorly organized in another, altering both absorption and the composition of material that continues through the gut.

Motility reflects these upstream differences. When material is properly prepared, the digestive tract can move it through in coordinated patterns that maximize mixing and contact with absorptive surfaces. When preparation is incomplete, motility becomes adaptive. The system may slow transit to allow more time for breakdown, increasing retention and fermentation, or accelerate transit to move unstable material through more quickly, reducing absorption. These patterns are not fixed. They shift with the state of the system, which is why an individual can experience alternating symptoms without any meaningful change in diet.

This variability creates the impression that certain foods are inconsistent or that reactions are unpredictable. In reality, the variability is structured. It follows the condition of the system at the time the food is processed. A meal consumed under conditions that support digestion is likely to be handled with minimal disturbance. The same meal consumed under conditions that suppress digestion produces a different outcome because the sequence begins from a reduced baseline. The input is constant, but the system is not.

Understanding digestion as state-dependent removes the need to attribute variability to the food. It shifts attention to the conditions under which the system is operating. When those conditions are stabilized, digestive output becomes more consistent. Acid production, enzyme release, bile flow, and motility begin to align with the demands of incoming material, and the system produces predictable results from the same inputs. Variability decreases not because the diet has been simplified, but because the system processing that diet is no longer fluctuating between states that support or suppress its function.

Why Food Quality Cannot Override Suppressed Physiology

Food quality determines the potential value of an input, but it does not determine whether that value is realized. The digestive system must convert structure into absorbable components before any nutrient can be used. When physiology is suppressed, that conversion is incomplete. High-quality inputs enter the system with intact structure, and if the machinery that alters that structure is operating below capacity, the outcome is constrained regardless of the starting material. The system cannot extract what it cannot process.

Suppression begins at the level of control and propagates through every stage of digestion. Reduced parasympathetic signaling lowers gastric acid output, which limits the unfolding of protein and the activation of enzymes that depend on an acidic environment. Pancreatic secretion becomes inconsistent, reducing the availability of proteases, lipases, and amylases at the moment they are needed. Bile release loses coordination with fat intake, leaving lipids in larger, less organized forms that resist absorption. Blood flow to the gastrointestinal tract decreases, limiting both secretion and the capacity of the intestinal lining to transport nutrients. These changes alter the system's ability to perform the transformations required to turn food into usable material.

Under these conditions, improving food quality changes the input but not the processing environment. A nutrient-dense meal still requires acid to denature proteins, enzymes to cleave macromolecules, and bile to emulsify fats. If those steps are incomplete, the material moves forward in a partially processed state. Larger fragments persist in the intestinal lumen, altering fluid balance and motility, and increasing the availability of substrates for microbial fermentation. The system is then forced to manage the consequences of incomplete breakdown rather than benefiting from the potential value of the food. The difference between high-quality and low-quality inputs becomes less relevant when both are processed under the same constraint.

This explains why individuals can adopt increasingly refined diets without resolving symptoms. Removing processed foods or selecting nutrient-dense options can reduce certain burdens, but it does not restore the outputs required for full digestion. The system remains limited by its capacity to generate acid, enzymes, and bile in the correct sequence. As long as that limitation persists, the range of foods that can be processed without disturbance remains narrow. The appearance of improvement reflects reduced demand on the system, not an increase in its functional capability.

The constraint also affects absorption and distribution. Even when some breakdown occurs, reduced blood flow and altered membrane transport limit how effectively nutrients move into circulation. Lipids that are not properly emulsified fail to form transport structures that can cross the intestinal lining. Amino acids derived from incomplete protein digestion are absorbed less efficiently and may appear in imbalanced patterns. Fat-soluble vitamins depend on bile-mediated transport and are directly affected by disruptions in lipid processing. The system does not selectively fail at one nutrient. It alters the entire flow of material from the lumen into the body.

Restoring physiology changes the outcome without requiring perfect inputs. When acid production reaches effective levels, protein structure is altered early and consistently. When enzyme release is synchronized with incoming material, macromolecules are reduced to absorbable units before they reach the distal intestine. When bile flow is coordinated, lipids are organized into structures that can be transported across membranes. Blood flow supports both secretion and absorption, allowing the system to move nutrients into circulation efficiently. Under these conditions, the system can extract value from a broader range of inputs because the transformations required to access that value are being completed.

Food quality matters once the system can process it. Without that capacity, quality remains potential rather than realized function. The limiting factor is not what is consumed, but whether the system can perform the sequence required to convert that input into structure and energy.

Chapter 2

Pace and Nervous System Control

The speed at which food is consumed alters the state of the nervous system, and that state determines how much of the digestive sequence is allowed to operate. Eating is not just the delivery of material into the gut. It is a signal that either permits or constrains the system that processes that material. When pace is rapid, the body interprets the environment as unstable or urgent, and sympathetic activity rises. This shifts control away from digestion and reduces the output of acid, enzymes, and bile before the system has had time to prepare. When pace is slower and controlled, parasympathetic signaling increases, and the system is given the conditions required to initiate digestion with sufficient output. The difference is established before the stomach receives the first portion of food.

Rapid intake compresses the preparatory phase into a narrow window that the system cannot fully utilize. Sensory input from taste, smell, and texture is reduced because food is moved quickly through the mouth, limiting the activation of neural pathways that prime gastric secretion. Salivary output decreases, and mechanical breakdown is incomplete. Larger particles enter the stomach, increasing the workload required for chemical processing. At the same time, the stomach has not yet increased acid production to levels that can compensate for this additional demand. The sequence begins with a mismatch between input and capacity, and that mismatch propagates through the rest of the system.

Gastric function is directly affected by this compression. Acid secretion depends on both anticipatory signaling and continued neural input during eating. When pace is rapid, the stomach receives a larger volume of material before acid output has reached effective levels. Proteins are exposed to a higher pH environment and remain partially folded. The stomach may respond by delaying emptying to allow more time for processing, which increases retention and the likelihood of fermentation. In other cases, material is passed forward before it has been adequately prepared, shifting the burden to the small intestine. Both outcomes reflect the same constraint. The stomach was not given the time or signaling required to match output to input.

Pancreatic and biliary responses are similarly affected. Enzyme release and bile flow are coordinated with the arrival of partially processed material from the stomach. When large volumes of inadequately prepared food enter the small intestine quickly, this coordination is disrupted. Enzymes may be insufficient relative to the load, and bile release may not align with the presence of dietary fat. Lipids remain in larger, less organized forms, and proteins and carbohydrates are not fully reduced. The intestine is forced to handle material that exceeds its optimal processing range, leading to changes in motility, fluid balance, and microbial activity.

Pace also influences motility through its effect on neural control. Rapid eating is associated with irregular contraction patterns that reduce the efficiency of mixing and propulsion. The system may alternate between slowed and accelerated transit as it attempts to manage the incoming material. Slowed transit increases retention and fermentation, while accelerated transit reduces absorption and increases variability in nutrient delivery. These patterns are not fixed but reflect the system's attempt to compensate for the initial mismatch created by rapid intake.

Over time, consistently rapid eating trains the system into a constrained operating mode. The nervous system begins to associate food intake with a state that suppresses digestive output. Baseline secretion decreases, and coordination between organs weakens. The system adapts to processing food under these conditions, but the adaptation reduces overall capacity. Symptoms become more consistent because the system is consistently starting from a reduced baseline.

Slowing the pace of eating changes the system before it changes the food. Extended sensory exposure increases parasympathetic signaling, allowing salivary secretion, gastric acid production, and anticipatory enzyme release to rise before the stomach receives a significant load.

Mechanical breakdown improves, reducing the size of particles that require chemical processing. The stomach is able to match acid output to incoming material, and the sequence begins with a more favorable alignment between input and capacity. Downstream processes then operate on substrates that have been properly prepared, reducing the need for compensation.

Pace is not a minor behavioral detail. It is a control variable that sets the operating conditions of the digestive system. When pace supports parasympathetic dominance, the sequence can proceed with the timing and output required for complete transformation. When pace reinforces sympathetic dominance, the system begins under constraint and carries that constraint through every stage. The outcome is determined less by what is eaten and more by the conditions under which the system is asked to process it.

Rushed Eating and Sequence Disruption

Rushed eating compresses the early stages of digestion into a time window that is too short for the system to prepare itself, and that compression alters the entire sequence that follows. Digestion depends on ordered transformations that begin before food reaches the stomach. Sensory input from chewing, taste, and smell activates neural pathways that increase salivary flow, initiate gastric acid production, and coordinate downstream secretion. When food is consumed quickly, this preparatory phase is truncated. The system receives volume before it has generated the output required to process that volume, and the sequence begins with a deficit that cannot be corrected later.

Mechanical breakdown is the first point of disruption. Inadequate chewing leaves food in larger particles with less surface area exposed to digestive fluids. These particles enter the stomach requiring more intensive chemical processing at a time when acid production has not yet reached effective levels. The stomach is forced to operate on material that is both structurally intact and poorly timed relative to its own secretory capacity. Proteins are not fully unfolded, and the initial transformation that enables enzymatic access is incomplete. The material that exits the stomach carries this structural resistance forward, increasing the burden on the small intestine.

Gastric timing becomes unstable under these conditions. The stomach must choose between delaying emptying to compensate for incomplete processing or moving material forward to prevent excessive retention.

Delayed emptying increases the opportunity for fermentation and pressure buildup, while accelerated emptying transfers inadequately prepared material into the intestine. Both outcomes originate from the same disruption. The stomach did not receive sufficient time or signaling to align acid output with incoming food. The sequence loses synchronization at its first major processing step.

Downstream systems inherit this mismatch. Pancreatic enzymes are released based on signals that assume a certain level of preparation has already occurred. When that preparation is incomplete, enzyme activity is less effective because substrates remain structurally resistant. Bile release may not align with the arrival of dietary fats, leaving lipids insufficiently emulsified and difficult to absorb. The small intestine receives material that exceeds its optimal processing range, and it responds by altering motility and fluid balance. Segmentation becomes less efficient, and peristalsis may either slow to allow more time for breakdown or accelerate to clear material that is not being handled effectively.

This disruption extends into the microbial environment. Larger, partially processed substrates provide a greater supply of fermentable material, increasing gas production and altering the composition of microbial activity. The intestine is exposed to compounds that would not be present in significant amounts if upstream processing were complete. These changes feed back into motility and barrier function, increasing variability in symptoms and reducing overall stability. What appears as bloating, discomfort, or irregularity is the downstream expression of a sequence that began without proper alignment.

Rushed eating does not simply reduce efficiency at one point. It shifts the entire system into a pattern of compensation. Each stage adjusts to the deficiencies of the previous one, but those adjustments introduce new constraints that propagate forward. Over time, this pattern can become habitual, lowering baseline output and weakening coordination between organs. The system becomes accustomed to operating under conditions where preparation is incomplete and timing is inconsistent.

Restoring sequence integrity requires restoring the conditions that allow preparation to occur before volume arrives. Slower eating increases sensory exposure, strengthens neural signaling, and allows secretory output to rise in advance of gastric loading. Mechanical breakdown improves, reducing the demand placed on chemical processing.

The stomach can align acid production with incoming material, and downstream systems receive substrates that have been properly prepared. The sequence stabilizes because each step is given the conditions required to perform its role before the next begins.

Training the Nervous System into Constrained Digestion

The nervous system does not treat each meal as an isolated event. It adapts to repeated patterns and establishes a baseline state that reflects how digestion is usually performed. When food is consistently consumed under conditions that suppress parasympathetic activity, the system learns to associate eating with reduced output. This is not a conscious process. It is a gradual recalibration of neural signaling that lowers secretory capacity, disrupts timing, and weakens coordination between digestive organs. What begins as a temporary constraint becomes the default operating mode.

This training occurs through repetition of mismatched input and state. When meals are eaten quickly, under stress, or without sufficient sensory engagement, the nervous system does not fully activate the pathways that drive digestion. Acid production remains lower, enzyme release is less synchronized, and bile flow becomes inconsistent. The system processes food under these conditions and adapts to make that constrained processing more stable. Over time, glands reduce their baseline output because they are not being regularly stimulated to operate at higher levels. The system becomes efficient at functioning within a limited range, but that efficiency comes at the cost of overall capacity.

Gastric function reflects this adaptation clearly. Acid secretion is not only a response to immediate signals but also a function of baseline readiness. When the stomach is repeatedly asked to process food with reduced neural input, its capacity to generate strong acid responses declines. Proteins are routinely exposed to suboptimal acidity, and the system normalizes this level of processing. Downstream organs adjust accordingly. The pancreas releases enzymes into an environment where substrates are not fully prepared, and the intestine develops motility patterns that attempt to manage partially processed material. The entire sequence shifts to accommodate the initial constraint.

This adaptation extends beyond secretion into timing and coordination. The precise alignment between stomach emptying, enzyme release, and bile flow depends on consistent signaling patterns. When those patterns are repeatedly disrupted, the synchronization between organs weakens. Enzymes may be released too early or too late relative to incoming material, and bile may not be delivered in a way that supports effective fat emulsification. The system continues to function, but it does so with reduced precision, increasing variability in outcomes and lowering the threshold for disruption.

The result is a system that appears sensitive and inconsistent, but is actually operating according to a learned pattern. Foods that require higher processing capacity produce symptoms because the system has been trained to operate below that capacity. Even when conditions improve temporarily, the underlying baseline remains constrained, and the system returns to its habitual mode of operation. This creates the impression that improvements are short-lived or dependent on strict control of inputs.

Reversing this pattern requires retraining the nervous system through repeated exposure to conditions that support full digestive output. Slower eating, consistent sensory engagement, and reduced sympathetic activation provide the signals required to increase parasympathetic tone. As these signals are repeated, secretory glands begin to increase baseline output, and coordination between organs improves. The system relearns how to initiate digestion with sufficient capacity and proper timing. This process does not occur instantly. It reflects the same adaptive mechanisms that created the constraint, but in the opposite direction.

As the nervous system shifts, the entire sequence begins to reorganize. The stomach produces stronger acid responses, enzymes are released in alignment with incoming material, and bile flow becomes more consistent. Motility stabilizes because the system is no longer compensating for incomplete preparation. The digestive process becomes more predictable because it is being driven by a control state that supports full function rather than limiting it.

Long-Term Cost of Speed on Digestion

Consistently eating at high speed does not just disrupt individual meals. It reshapes the baseline performance of the digestive system over time. The body adapts to the conditions it is repeatedly exposed to, and when those conditions involve compressed eating, reduced sensory engagement, and elevated sympathetic activity, the system recalibrates toward lower output and weaker coordination. What begins as a temporary mismatch between input and processing capacity becomes a stable operating pattern in which digestion is routinely initiated under constraint.

The first cost appears at the level of secretion. Gastric acid production is driven by neural signaling that reflects both immediate input and habitual patterns. When meals are repeatedly consumed quickly, the preparatory phase is shortened, and the stomach is not consistently stimulated to reach higher levels of acid output. Over time, this reduces baseline acid capacity. Proteins are exposed to a less acidic environment, and the initial transformation that enables enzymatic access becomes incomplete by default. The pancreas then releases enzymes into a system where substrates are not fully prepared, lowering the efficiency of breakdown and increasing the amount of partially processed material that moves into the intestine.

Bile dynamics are also affected. Rapid intake disrupts the timing signals that coordinate gallbladder contraction with the arrival of dietary fat. When this pattern is repeated, bile release becomes less precise, and fats are not consistently emulsified into structures that can be absorbed efficiently. Lipids pass through the small intestine in larger, less organized forms, altering both nutrient absorption and the composition of material that reaches the colon. This shift changes the internal environment, increasing reliance on microbial processing of substrates that should have been handled earlier in the sequence.

Motility adapts in response to these upstream inefficiencies. When the system is consistently presented with inadequately prepared material, it develops patterns that attempt to manage that condition. Transit may slow to allow more time for breakdown, leading to increased retention and fermentation, or it may accelerate to clear material that cannot be processed effectively, reducing absorption. These patterns can alternate because the system is not stable. It is responding to variable levels of incomplete processing. Over time, this variability becomes more pronounced, and digestive outcomes become less predictable.

The intestinal barrier is exposed to a higher load of partially processed fragments as this pattern continues. Larger molecules that would normally be reduced earlier in the sequence interact with the lining of the intestine, increasing the likelihood of immune activation. This does not occur as a primary dysfunction but as a response to material that has not been properly prepared. The immune system adjusts to this increased exposure, and inflammatory signaling becomes more frequent.

This adds another layer of instability, as immune activity feeds back into motility, secretion, and neural signaling.

Energy extraction becomes less reliable as well. Incomplete breakdown and inconsistent absorption lead to fluctuations in nutrient availability. Amino acids may be delivered in uneven patterns, fats may not be fully absorbed, and fat-soluble vitamins depend on bile-mediated transport that is no longer consistent. The system continues to receive input, but the conversion of that input into usable material becomes variable. This variability extends beyond the digestive tract, affecting systemic processes that rely on steady nutrient delivery.

These changes do not occur abruptly. They accumulate through repetition. Each meal consumed under constrained conditions reinforces the same pattern, gradually lowering capacity and weakening coordination. The system becomes efficient at operating within these limits, but that efficiency masks a reduction in overall function. Foods that once required minimal effort to process begin to produce symptoms because the system is no longer capable of completing the sequence at the required level.

Reversing the long-term cost of speed requires restoring the conditions that allow full engagement of the digestive system. Slowing the pace of eating reintroduces the preparatory phase, increases parasympathetic signaling, and allows secretion to rise before the stomach receives a significant load. As this pattern is repeated, baseline output begins to increase, and coordination between organs improves. The system gradually shifts back toward a state where each stage prepares the next, reducing the need for compensation and restoring stability across the entire sequence.

Calm Eating as Capacity Restoration

Calm eating alters the control layer that determines how much of the digestive system is allowed to operate, and this change in control increases capacity across the entire sequence. When the body enters a state that supports parasympathetic activity, secretory output rises, timing between organs becomes more precise, and blood flow is directed toward the gastrointestinal tract. These changes are not superficial. They directly affect the system's ability to perform the transformations required to convert food into absorbable material. Capacity increases because the system is no longer operating under constraint.

The preparatory phase expands under calm conditions. Sensory exposure to food is extended, allowing neural signaling to build before a significant volume reaches the stomach. Salivary secretion increases, initiating early enzymatic activity and improving mechanical breakdown through more effective chewing. Particles entering the stomach are smaller and more uniform, reducing the demand placed on gastric processing. At the same time, gastric glands are activated in advance, and acid production begins to rise before the first substantial input arrives. The system aligns output with incoming material instead of reacting after the fact.

Gastric function improves as a result of this alignment. Acid levels reach the threshold required to alter protein structure consistently, exposing peptide bonds for enzymatic cleavage. The stomach is able to process material efficiently without relying on prolonged retention or premature emptying. The material that exits the stomach is chemically prepared for the next stage, reducing the burden placed on the small intestine. This shift at the first major processing step propagates forward, improving the efficiency of the entire sequence.

Pancreatic and biliary responses become more coordinated when the system is operating under calm conditions. Enzyme release is synchronized with the arrival of partially processed material, allowing macromolecules to be reduced to absorbable units before they move deeper into the intestine. Bile flow aligns with the presence of dietary fat, organizing lipids into emulsified structures that can be transported across the intestinal lining. These processes depend on timing as much as on quantity. Calm eating restores that timing, allowing each stage to prepare the next with greater precision.

Motility stabilizes because the system is no longer compensating for incomplete preparation. Coordinated contractions mix and propel material in patterns that maximize contact with digestive surfaces without excessive retention or premature transit. The intestine receives substrates that are closer to their absorbable form, reducing the need to adjust transit speed in response to poorly processed material. This stability extends to the microbial environment, where reduced availability of large, fermentable substrates decreases gas production and variability in internal conditions.

Repeated exposure to calm eating conditions retrains the nervous system and increases baseline capacity. Secretory glands respond to consistent stimulation by increasing output, and coordination between organs becomes more reliable. The system begins to initiate digestion from a higher starting point, reducing the likelihood that any given meal will exceed its processing limits. Foods that previously required restriction can be handled with less disruption because the system has regained the ability to complete the required transformations.

Capacity restoration through calm eating does not rely on altering the food itself. It relies on restoring the conditions under which the system operates. As parasympathetic signaling becomes more consistent, the digestive sequence regains its structure. Each stage performs its role with sufficient output and timing, and the system transitions from compensation to coordinated function.

Why Early Focus Should Be State, Not Food

The first constraint on digestion is not the composition of the meal but the condition of the system that receives it. If the control layer is set to suppression, every downstream process begins below capacity. Acid output is reduced, enzymes are released with poor timing, bile flow loses alignment with fat intake, and blood is diverted away from the gut. Under these conditions, even simple inputs arrive at each stage in a partially prepared state. Changing the food does not correct this starting deficit. It only changes what is being processed under the same constraint.

State determines whether the sequence can initiate with sufficient output. When parasympathetic signaling is present, secretion increases before significant volume reaches the stomach, and the system aligns preparation with input. Proteins encounter an acidic environment that unfolds structure early, enzymes meet substrates that are accessible, and bile arrives when lipids require organization into transportable forms. When this state is absent, the system reacts after the fact. The stomach attempts to increase acid after material has already arrived, enzymes are released into an environment that has not been properly prepared, and bile flow may not match the presence of dietary fat. The sequence begins out of alignment, and that misalignment carries forward.

Focusing on food first reduces demand but does not restore capacity. Removing inputs that are difficult to process can lower symptom intensity because the system is no longer being pushed beyond its limits. The underlying outputs remain unchanged. Acid remains low, enzyme release remains inconsistent, and bile flow remains poorly timed. As long as these constraints persist, the range of tolerable foods stays narrow. Over time, the threshold for disruption can drop further because the system has not been trained to operate at higher capacity.

State-first correction changes the system before it changes the input. Increasing parasympathetic tone raises baseline secretion, improves coordination between organs, and directs blood flow toward the tissues responsible for processing and absorption. The same meal that previously exceeded the system's limits can now be handled because the transformations required to process it are being completed. Downstream variability decreases because material is no longer entering each stage in a compromised form.

This approach also stabilizes feedback. When the sequence operates with sufficient output, the signals that regulate motility, secretion, and absorption become more consistent. The intestine receives substrates that are closer to their absorbable form, reducing the need for compensatory changes in transit speed. Microbial activity shifts because less fermentable material is available. Immune exposure decreases as fewer large fragments reach the barrier. These changes emerge from restoring the starting conditions rather than from selecting a narrower set of inputs.

Prioritizing state establishes a foundation on which food quality can then have its intended effect. Once the system can perform the required transformations, differences in input composition begin to matter in a meaningful way. Nutrient density can be realized because nutrients are being fully extracted and transported. Without that foundation, quality remains unrealized potential. The system limits the outcome regardless of the input.

Early focus on state aligns intervention with the structure of digestion. It addresses the control layer that determines whether the sequence can operate at all. When that layer is restored, subsequent adjustments to food become additive rather than compensatory, and the system moves toward stable, predictable function.

PART II

THE MOUTH–BRAIN–GUT LOOP

Chapter 3

The Mouth as the First Organ of Digestion

Digestion begins in the mouth because the system requires early transformation and signaling before material reaches the stomach. The mouth is not a passive entry point. It is an active interface where mechanical reduction, fluid mixing, and neural activation converge to prepare the entire digestive tract for incoming food. What happens here determines how effectively the system can initiate the sequence that follows. When this stage is performed with sufficient engagement, downstream processes receive material that is already partially processed and a signal that digestion should proceed at full capacity. When it is bypassed or compressed, both the material and the signaling are degraded from the start.

Mechanical breakdown is the first transformation. Chewing reduces particle size and increases surface area, allowing digestive fluids to interact with food more effectively. Larger particles require more intensive chemical processing later, placing a greater demand on gastric acid and enzymatic activity. When chewing is thorough, the stomach receives material that is easier to penetrate and alter. This reduces the workload required to unfold protein structure and allows enzymatic processes to proceed more efficiently. Mechanical reduction is not separate from chemical digestion. It sets the conditions under which chemical digestion can occur.

Saliva introduces the first layer of chemical processing while also altering the physical properties of the food. It contains enzymes that begin the breakdown of certain macromolecules and fluids that hydrate and disperse particles into a cohesive mass. This hydration improves the ability of the stomach to mix and expose material to acid. Without sufficient saliva, food enters the stomach in a drier, less integrated form that resists uniform exposure to digestive fluids. The result is uneven processing, where some portions are altered effectively and others remain structurally intact.

The mouth also serves as a signaling center that activates the digestive system before swallowing occurs. Sensory input from taste, smell, and texture triggers neural pathways that increase salivary secretion, stimulate gastric acid production, and prepare the pancreas and liver for incoming material. This anticipatory phase allows the system to align output with input. When food reaches the stomach under these conditions, acid production is already increasing, and the system is positioned to begin chemical transformation immediately. When this signaling is weak or absent, the stomach must react after food has arrived, creating a delay that reduces the effectiveness of early processing.

The quality of this signaling depends on engagement within the mouth. Rapid eating, minimal chewing, and limited sensory exposure reduce the activation of these pathways. The system receives less information about the incoming material and generates a weaker preparatory response. This leads to lower acid output, less coordinated enzyme release, and reduced bile signaling. The sequence begins with a deficit that carries forward into every subsequent stage. The stomach becomes a reactive environment rather than a prepared one, and downstream processes are forced to compensate.

Swallowing marks the transition from preparation to processing, but the quality of that transition is determined by what occurred in the mouth. A well-formed bolus, adequately hydrated and mechanically reduced, moves into the stomach as a substrate that can be efficiently transformed. A poorly prepared bolus arrives as a collection of larger, less integrated particles that require additional processing under conditions that may already be constrained. The difference at this stage influences the entire sequence, as each downstream step inherits the properties of the material it receives.

Treating the mouth as the first organ of digestion reframes the starting point of the system. It establishes that digestion does not begin in the stomach and that early-stage preparation is not optional. Mechanical breakdown, salivary processing, and neural activation form the initial conditions that determine how effectively the system can operate. When this stage is restored, the sequence begins with alignment between input and capacity, and the burden placed on downstream processes is reduced.

Cephalic Phase Activation

The cephalic phase is the initial activation of digestion driven by sensory input before food reaches the stomach. Sight, smell, taste, and even the expectation of eating trigger neural pathways that increase secretory output across the digestive system. This phase prepares the stomach, pancreas, and liver to receive incoming material by elevating acid production, priming enzyme release, and initiating signals that will coordinate bile flow. The system does not wait for food to arrive and then react. It anticipates and adjusts its output in advance, aligning capacity with the expected load.

This activation is mediated primarily through parasympathetic signaling. Sensory input is processed centrally and transmitted through pathways such as the vagus nerve to digestive organs, where it directly influences glandular activity. Gastric parietal cells begin increasing acid secretion, chief cells prepare to release enzymes, and the pancreas and gallbladder are primed for coordinated output. The result is a system that is already moving toward full operational capacity by the time swallowing occurs. The first material that enters the stomach encounters an environment that is prepared to alter its structure immediately.

The strength of this phase depends on the quality and duration of sensory exposure. Extended interaction with food in the mouth increases the intensity of neural signaling. Taste receptors are stimulated more fully, olfactory input remains active, and the mechanical act of chewing reinforces the signal that digestion is about to proceed. When this exposure is sufficient, acid production rises in parallel with intake, reducing the lag between arrival and processing. When exposure is brief, as in rapid eating, the signal is weaker and shorter. The stomach receives food before acid output has reached effective levels, and the sequence begins with reduced alignment between input and capacity.

The cephalic phase also influences downstream coordination. Signals generated at this stage contribute to the timing of pancreatic enzyme release and bile delivery. These processes are not isolated reactions but part of a coordinated sequence that begins with early activation. When the cephalic phase is strong, enzyme secretion and bile flow are more likely to align with the arrival of partially processed material from the stomach. When it is weak, these outputs become less synchronized, and the system loses precision. The small intestine receives material that has not been fully prepared and must operate under conditions that favor compensation rather than efficient processing.

Disruption of this phase does not eliminate digestion, but it lowers the starting point of the entire system. Each subsequent stage begins from a position of reduced output, and the effects accumulate. Proteins are not fully unfolded, enzymes encounter resistant substrates, fats are not consistently emulsified, and absorption becomes less efficient. These changes are often attributed to later stages, but they originate at the level of early activation. The sequence is misaligned from the beginning.

Restoring cephalic phase activation increases capacity before the first transformation occurs. Slower eating, thorough chewing, and sustained sensory engagement extend the duration and intensity of neural signaling, allowing secretory output to rise in advance. The stomach receives material under conditions that support immediate processing, and downstream systems operate on substrates that have been properly prepared. The sequence regains alignment because the system has been activated before it is asked to perform.

Sensory Signaling and Digestive Preparation

Sensory input sets the initial conditions for digestion by informing the system that food is about to enter and by specifying the type of material that will need to be processed. Taste, smell, texture, and visual cues activate neural pathways that increase secretory output and coordinate timing across digestive organs. This signaling occurs before swallowing and establishes the level of readiness within the system. When it is strong, the stomach begins increasing acid production, the pancreas prepares for enzyme release, and bile flow is primed to align with incoming fat. The system does not wait for physical contact with food in the stomach to begin these processes. It prepares in advance so that the first stage of chemical transformation can occur immediately.

The intensity and duration of this signaling depend on engagement within the mouth. Prolonged exposure to taste and texture provides continuous input that reinforces neural activation. Chewing extends this exposure, allowing signals to build rather than peak briefly and decline. As this occurs, salivary secretion increases, and early enzymatic activity begins to alter certain components of the food. More importantly, the central control of digestion adjusts its output upward, ensuring that gastric and pancreatic responses are scaled to match the anticipated load. When sensory engagement is limited, these signals are reduced. The system receives less information and generates a weaker preparatory response, leading to lower output at the start of digestion.

This preparation directly affects the efficiency of gastric processing. When sensory signaling is sufficient, the stomach receives food under conditions where acid production is already rising. Proteins encounter an environment capable of altering their structure early, which facilitates subsequent enzymatic breakdown. When signaling is weak, acid output lags behind the arrival of food. The stomach must increase secretion after material has already entered, creating a delay that reduces the effectiveness of the initial transformation. The material that leaves the stomach reflects this delay, carrying more structural resistance into the small intestine.

Pancreatic and biliary coordination also depend on early signaling. The release of enzymes and bile is timed based on input that begins in the cephalic phase. When this input is strong, enzyme secretion aligns with the arrival of partially processed material, and bile is delivered in a pattern that supports fat emulsification. When input is weak, these processes lose synchronization. Enzymes may be released in insufficient amounts or at the wrong time, and bile may not be available when fats require organization into absorbable structures. The system continues to function, but it does so with reduced precision and increased variability.

Sensory signaling therefore acts as a control input that determines how the sequence of digestion is initiated. It does not change the composition of the food, but it changes the system's ability to process that composition. Strong signaling creates alignment between input and capacity, allowing each stage to operate with sufficient output and timing. Weak signaling lowers the starting point of the sequence, forcing downstream systems to compensate for incomplete preparation. The difference in outcome is established before the stomach begins its work, based on how effectively the system was prepared to receive what is about to arrive.

Mechanical Breakdown and Signaling Integration

Mechanical breakdown in the mouth is not a separate step from chemical digestion. It is the first transformation that determines how effectively all subsequent transformations can occur, and it operates in parallel with neural signaling that prepares the rest of the system.

Chewing reduces particle size, increases surface area, and distributes saliva throughout the food matrix, but at the same time it amplifies sensory input that drives parasympathetic activation. The physical act of breaking down food and the neural signaling that coordinates digestion are integrated processes. When one is reduced, the other is weakened, and the sequence begins with both structural and signaling deficits.

Particle size directly affects how digestive fluids interact with food. Smaller, well-chewed particles expose more surface area to gastric acid, allowing proteins to be unfolded more uniformly and efficiently. Larger particles resist penetration, leaving internal portions structurally intact even as outer layers are partially processed. This creates uneven substrates that move through the system with variable levels of preparation. Enzymes encounter these substrates with reduced efficiency because access to cleavage sites is inconsistent. Mechanical reduction in the mouth determines whether the stomach is working on a uniform substrate or a fragmented one with areas that remain resistant to change.

Saliva integrates into this process by hydrating and dispersing particles into a cohesive bolus. This hydration allows gastric mixing to occur more effectively, ensuring that acid can contact the entire mass rather than isolated regions. Without sufficient saliva, food enters the stomach in a drier, less integrated form that limits uniform exposure to digestive fluids. Some portions may be adequately processed while others remain largely unchanged, increasing the variability of material that moves forward. The stomach must then compensate for this inconsistency, often by prolonging retention or passing partially processed material into the intestine.

At the same time, chewing reinforces sensory signaling that drives digestive preparation. Each cycle of mastication stimulates taste receptors, maintains olfactory input, and sends continuous feedback to the central nervous system. This sustained input increases parasympathetic signaling, which in turn elevates gastric acid production and primes pancreatic and biliary output. Mechanical breakdown therefore functions as a driver of signaling intensity. The longer and more thoroughly food is processed in the mouth, the stronger the preparatory response becomes. When chewing is minimal, both the physical reduction of food and the signaling required to prepare the system are diminished simultaneously.

This integration affects the timing of the entire sequence. When mechanical breakdown and signaling are aligned, the stomach receives a well-prepared bolus under conditions where acid production is already increasing. The initial transformation occurs without delay, and downstream processes receive substrates that have been uniformly altered. When this alignment is absent, the stomach must process larger, less hydrated particles while also increasing acid output after the fact. The sequence begins out of sync, and that misalignment propagates through enzyme release, bile flow, and intestinal absorption.

Mechanical breakdown and signaling integration establish the first level of coordination in digestion. They determine both the structural state of the incoming material and the readiness of the system that will process it. When this stage is executed with sufficient engagement, the system begins with alignment between input and capacity. When it is reduced, the system starts with uneven substrates and weakened signaling, forcing every downstream step to compensate for conditions that should have been resolved at the beginning.

Chapter 4

Early-Phase Digestive Signaling

Early-phase digestive signaling establishes the operating conditions for the entire system before the stomach begins its primary work. This phase extends beyond the mouth and into the initial interaction between the stomach and the upper small intestine, where neural and hormonal signals coordinate secretion, motility, and timing across multiple organs. The system uses this early window to align output with the nature and volume of incoming material. When this signaling is intact, digestion proceeds with coordinated precision. When it is weak or disordered, the sequence begins out of alignment and every downstream process operates under constraint.

The stomach is not only a processing chamber but also a signaling hub. As food enters, mechanoreceptors and chemoreceptors detect volume, composition, and physical properties. These signals are transmitted through neural pathways and local reflexes that adjust acid secretion, enzyme release, and the rate of gastric emptying. Protein content, fat presence, and overall load influence how strongly these responses are activated. When early-phase signaling is functioning properly, the stomach modulates its output to match the demands of the meal, increasing acid for protein-rich inputs and adjusting emptying to ensure that material is adequately prepared before entering the small intestine.

Hormonal signaling reinforces and extends this coordination. Cells in the stomach and upper intestine release messengers that regulate downstream activity based on what has been detected upstream. These signals influence pancreatic enzyme secretion, gallbladder contraction, and intestinal motility. They create a feedback loop that links the stomach to the small intestine, ensuring that each stage is informed about the state of the material it will receive. When this communication is precise, enzyme release and bile flow are timed to coincide with the arrival of partially processed material, allowing breakdown and absorption to proceed efficiently.

The timing of gastric emptying is a critical component of this phase. The stomach does not release its contents at a fixed rate. It adjusts emptying based on how well the material has been processed and how prepared the small intestine is to receive it. When early signaling is intact, this timing is synchronized. The intestine receives material in controlled amounts that match its capacity for enzymatic breakdown and absorption. When signaling is disrupted, this synchronization breaks down. The stomach may release material too quickly, overwhelming the intestine with inadequately prepared substrates, or hold material too long, increasing retention and altering internal conditions.

This phase also determines how effectively fats are handled. The presence of lipids triggers signals that coordinate bile release and pancreatic lipase activity. These signals originate early and depend on accurate detection of fat content. When signaling is strong, bile is delivered in a pattern that allows lipids to be emulsified into structures that can be absorbed. When signaling is weak or mistimed, bile release may be insufficient or delayed, leaving fats in forms that resist transport across the intestinal lining. This alters both nutrient absorption and the composition of material that continues through the gut.

Disruption in early-phase signaling often originates from deficiencies in the stages that precede it. Weak sensory activation, rapid eating, and suppressed parasympathetic tone reduce the strength of the initial signals that drive this phase. As a result, the stomach and intestine operate with incomplete information and reduced coordination. Each organ continues to function, but the system as a whole loses synchronization. The material that moves through the sequence is processed under conditions that vary from one stage to the next, increasing inefficiency and variability in outcomes.

Restoring early-phase signaling requires strengthening the inputs that initiate it and re-establishing the conditions that allow it to operate. When sensory engagement is sufficient, parasympathetic signaling is present, and mechanical preparation in the mouth is adequate, the stomach receives clear and sustained signals about incoming material.

Hormonal and neural pathways then coordinate downstream responses with greater precision. The sequence begins with alignment, allowing each stage to prepare the next without relying on compensation.

Saliva, Enzymes, and Anticipatory Signaling

Saliva initiates digestion by combining early chemical breakdown with a signaling function that prepares the rest of the system for incoming material. As food enters the mouth, salivary glands increase output under parasympathetic control, delivering fluid, electrolytes, and enzymes that begin to act on specific components of the meal. This activity is modest in terms of total breakdown, but it establishes the first chemical interaction between food and the body. At the same time, the presence of saliva and the act of chewing amplify neural signaling that raises gastric and pancreatic output in advance of swallowing. The system is not waiting to react. It is scaling its activity based on what is being sensed.

Salivary enzymes begin the reduction of certain macromolecules while food is still in the mouth. This early activity alters the physical structure of the bolus and creates gradients that continue to influence processing after swallowing. Hydration from saliva disperses particles and reduces friction, allowing gastric mixing to occur more uniformly. A well-hydrated bolus exposes more surface area to acid and enzymes once it reaches the stomach. When saliva is limited, food enters in a drier, less integrated form that resists uniform exposure to digestive fluids. Portions of the meal may be processed effectively while others remain structurally intact, creating variability that persists downstream.

The signaling role of saliva is tied to its method of release. Salivary secretion is driven by neural pathways that also regulate gastric acid production and pancreatic enzyme release. As salivation increases, it reflects an increase in parasympathetic activity that extends beyond the mouth. This coordinated activation raises acid output in the stomach and primes the pancreas to deliver enzymes in alignment with incoming material. The system uses salivation as both a functional and informational signal. It indicates that digestion is about to proceed and adjusts downstream output accordingly.

Anticipatory signaling extends this coordination further. Sensory input from taste and smell is integrated with the act of chewing to generate a sustained neural signal that informs the system about the composition and volume of the meal. This information influences not only how much acid and enzyme will be produced, but also when they will be released. The timing established during this phase determines whether gastric and intestinal processes will align with the arrival of food. When signaling is strong, acid production rises before significant gastric loading occurs, and enzyme release is synchronized with the movement of partially processed material into the small intestine. When signaling is weak, these processes lag, and the sequence begins with misalignment.

This early phase shapes the efficiency of every subsequent stage. Proper salivary function and anticipatory signaling reduce the burden on gastric processing by delivering a bolus that is both mechanically and chemically prepared. They also ensure that downstream systems are operating at a level that matches the demands of the meal. When this phase is reduced, the system must compensate later. The stomach attempts to increase acid after the fact, enzymes are released into an environment that has not been properly prepared, and bile flow may not align with fat intake. These compensations increase variability and reduce overall efficiency.

Saliva, enzymes, and anticipatory signaling therefore establish the initial conditions for digestion. They determine both the structure of the material entering the stomach and the readiness of the system that will process it. When this phase is intact, the sequence begins with alignment between input and capacity. When it is weakened, the system starts with deficits that propagate through every stage, increasing the likelihood of incomplete transformation and downstream instability.

Brain–Gut Coordination Before Swallowing

Coordination between the brain and the digestive tract is established before food leaves the mouth, and this coordination determines how effectively the system will handle what follows. The act of chewing and sensing food generates continuous neural input that is integrated centrally and transmitted to the stomach, pancreas, liver, and intestine. This input does not simply signal that food is present. It carries information about volume, texture, and composition, allowing the system to scale its output in advance. By the time swallowing occurs, multiple organs have already adjusted their activity to match what is about to arrive.

The vagal pathway serves as the primary conduit for this coordination. Signals generated in response to sensory input increase parasympathetic tone, which raises gastric acid production, primes enzyme release, and prepares bile delivery. These changes occur while food is still in the mouth. The stomach begins increasing its secretory activity, the pancreas adjusts its readiness to release enzymes, and the gallbladder is signaled to prepare for contraction. The system is aligning its capacity with the anticipated load so that the first stage of processing can occur without delay.

This coordination also influences how the stomach will manage incoming material. Neural input from the cephalic phase affects both secretion and motility, determining how strongly the stomach will contract and how quickly it will empty its contents. When signaling is sufficient, the stomach is prepared to both chemically and mechanically process food as it arrives. When signaling is weak, the stomach receives material without having increased its output, and it must attempt to compensate after the fact. This delay alters the initial transformation and affects the quality of material that moves forward.

The pancreas and liver are integrated into this early coordination through the same signaling network. Enzyme secretion and bile release depend on timing that is established before swallowing. When the brain–gut connection is active, these organs are primed to respond in synchrony with the movement of food from the stomach into the small intestine. This synchronization ensures that macromolecules are reduced efficiently and that lipids are emulsified at the moment they require it. When coordination is reduced, these responses become mistimed, and the system loses precision.

The strength of this coordination depends on the continuity of sensory input. Sustained chewing and engagement maintain the signal, allowing output to rise progressively. Rapid intake interrupts this process, shortening the duration of signaling and reducing its intensity. The system receives a weaker preparatory signal and begins digestion from a lower baseline. Each downstream stage is then forced to operate with reduced input, increasing the likelihood of incomplete processing.

Brain–gut coordination before swallowing establishes the timing and scale of the digestive sequence. It determines whether the system will begin with aligned output or with a deficit that must be managed later. When this coordination is intact, the transition from preparation to processing occurs without interruption, and each organ contributes at the appropriate moment. When it is weakened, the sequence begins out of sync, and the effects propagate through every stage of digestion.

How Weak Signaling Propagates Downstream

Weak early-phase signaling lowers the starting output of the entire digestive system, and that deficit carries forward through each stage as a compounding constraint. When sensory input and parasympathetic activation are insufficient, gastric secretion begins below the level required to alter incoming material effectively. Acid production rises slowly and often remains suboptimal relative to the volume and composition of the meal. Proteins enter an environment that does not fully unfold their structure, leaving peptide bonds less accessible to enzymatic cleavage. The stomach still mixes and churns, but the chemical conditions required for uniform transformation are not established early enough.

This initial deficit changes the form of material that exits the stomach. Instead of a consistently processed mixture, the small intestine receives substrates with uneven levels of preparation. Some fractions are partially broken down while others retain structural resistance. Pancreatic enzymes encounter this variability and must operate on substrates that are not uniformly accessible. Enzyme activity depends on contact with specific sites, and when those sites are hidden within intact structures, breakdown slows. The intestine compensates by extending exposure time or increasing secretory output where possible, but this compensation is inconsistent and often incomplete.

Bile coordination is affected in parallel. Early signaling contributes to the timing of bile release, aligning it with the arrival of lipids that require emulsification. When signaling is weak, this timing shifts. Bile may be released in insufficient quantities or at points that do not match the presence of dietary fat. Lipids remain in larger aggregates that resist dispersion, reducing the efficiency of lipase activity and limiting the formation of transportable structures. As these partially processed fats move through the intestine, they alter the composition of the luminal environment and influence how other nutrients are handled.

Motility patterns adjust in response to this altered substrate. The intestine uses feedback from the material it receives to regulate transit speed. When substrates are inadequately processed, the system may slow movement to increase exposure time, or in some cases accelerate transit if irritation or osmotic effects are present. These adjustments are reactive rather than coordinated. The sequence loses its predictable timing, and the relationship between secretion, breakdown, and absorption becomes less stable. Variability increases from one meal to the next because the starting conditions are inconsistent.

Absorption efficiency declines as a direct consequence of these upstream changes. Nutrients that have not been reduced to their absorbable forms remain within the lumen, and the transport mechanisms of the intestinal lining are underutilized. Larger fragments and unprocessed components continue forward, increasing the load on distal regions of the gut. Microbial populations encounter substrates that would normally be absorbed earlier, shifting fermentation patterns and altering the chemical environment. This introduces additional variability and can amplify symptoms that are often attributed solely to microbial imbalance.

The propagation of weak signaling is therefore not a single failure but a sequence of dependent effects. A reduced signal at the beginning lowers acid output, which alters substrate structure, which affects enzyme efficiency, which disrupts bile coordination, which changes motility, which reduces absorption. Each step inherits the conditions created by the previous one. Strengthening the initial signal raises the starting output and changes the trajectory of the entire sequence, allowing each stage to operate on material that has been properly prepared and aligned with the system's capacity.

PART III

STOMACH AS THE PRIMARY PROCESSOR

Chapter 5

Stomach Acid and Protein Transformation

The stomach establishes the first major chemical transformation of food by creating an acidic environment that alters protein structure and sets the conditions for enzymatic breakdown. Acid is not a secondary component of digestion. It defines how proteins behave once they enter the system and determines whether downstream enzymes can access their targets. When acid output is sufficient, proteins lose their folded configuration, exposing internal bonds that can be cleaved efficiently. When acid is reduced or delayed, proteins retain structural resistance, and every subsequent stage is forced to operate on a substrate that has not been properly prepared.

Protein transformation in the stomach begins with denaturation. The acidic environment disrupts the forces that maintain protein folding, causing the structure to open and become more accessible. This change is required before proteolytic enzymes can act effectively. Enzymes do not break down intact, tightly folded proteins with the same efficiency as unfolded ones. Acid therefore functions as a structural modifier that prepares proteins for enzymatic cleavage. Without this step, enzymatic activity is limited by the physical configuration of the substrate rather than by enzyme availability alone.

Enzyme activation within the stomach depends on this acidic environment. Proteolytic enzymes are released in an inactive form and require low pH conditions to become active. When acid production is adequate, these enzymes are converted into their active state and begin cleaving peptide bonds, reducing large protein structures into smaller fragments. This process generates peptides that can be further processed in the small intestine. When acid levels are insufficient, enzyme activation is reduced, and the breakdown of proteins is incomplete. Larger fragments persist and move forward without having undergone the necessary initial reduction.

The timing of acid production is as important as its magnitude. When acid output rises before or as food enters the stomach, proteins are exposed to conditions that allow immediate denaturation and enzymatic action. When acid production lags, food accumulates in an environment that is not yet capable of effective transformation. The stomach attempts to increase acid after the fact, but the delay allows proteins to remain structurally intact for longer periods. This affects how thoroughly they are processed before leaving the stomach and alters the composition of material entering the small intestine.

Stomach acid also influences the physical behavior of the meal. It contributes to the breakdown of connective structures within food, facilitating mixing and allowing gastric motility to distribute contents more evenly. This uniformity ensures that enzymes can act across the entire mass rather than on isolated regions. When acid is low, mixing may still occur, but the structural integrity of food components is less affected, and uneven processing persists. Portions of the meal may be reduced effectively while others remain resistant, increasing variability in the substrate delivered downstream.

The consequences of impaired protein transformation extend beyond the stomach. The small intestine relies on receiving peptides that have already been partially reduced. Pancreatic enzymes are designed to act on these smaller fragments, completing the breakdown into absorbable amino acids. When larger, less processed proteins enter the intestine, enzyme efficiency decreases because access to cleavage sites is limited. The system compensates by increasing enzyme output or altering transit time, but these adjustments are not always sufficient to achieve complete breakdown.

Stomach acid therefore sets the trajectory for protein digestion. It determines whether proteins are structurally prepared for enzymatic reduction and whether enzymes can operate at full efficiency. Adequate acid output aligns the system so that each stage builds on the work of the previous one. Reduced or delayed acid output creates a starting deficit that propagates through the sequence, affecting enzyme activity, absorption, and the overall stability of digestion.

Acid as Structural Modifier

Acid in the stomach functions by changing the physical state of proteins rather than by breaking them down directly into absorbable units. The drop in pH alters charge distribution along amino acid side chains, disrupts hydrogen bonding, and weakens hydrophobic interactions that hold the folded structure together. As these stabilizing forces are reduced, proteins unfold and lose their compact configuration. This transition exposes internal peptide bonds that were previously inaccessible, converting a tightly organized structure into a more open substrate that enzymes can act upon.

This structural shift determines whether proteolytic enzymes can operate efficiently. Enzymes require access to specific regions of a protein in order to cleave peptide bonds. When proteins remain folded, many of these regions are buried within the interior of the molecule, limiting enzymatic contact. Acid-driven unfolding brings these regions to the surface, increasing the number of available cleavage sites. The rate of enzymatic breakdown is therefore governed by how completely this structural modification has occurred before enzymes begin acting. Without sufficient unfolding, enzyme presence alone does not translate into effective digestion.

The effect of acid extends beyond individual protein molecules to the larger architecture of the meal. Connective tissues and structural proteins within food matrices are altered by low pH, reducing their resistance to mechanical and enzymatic processing. This allows gastric motility to distribute contents more evenly and ensures that enzymes can interact with a more uniform substrate. When this modification is incomplete, portions of the meal retain structural integrity that resists both mixing and enzymatic access. The result is uneven processing, where some regions are reduced effectively while others persist in a more intact form.

Acid also establishes the conditions required for enzyme activation. Proteolytic enzymes released in the stomach depend on a low pH environment to convert into their active form. This creates a sequence in which structural modification and enzymatic activity are linked. Acid unfolds proteins and simultaneously activates the enzymes that will cleave them. When acid levels are sufficient, these processes occur in coordination, allowing transformation to proceed without interruption. When acid is reduced, both unfolding and enzyme activation are limited, and the system operates with diminished efficiency.

The timing of this structural modification influences how material is presented to the small intestine. When proteins are unfolded early, enzymatic cleavage progresses to a stage where smaller peptides are generated before gastric emptying. These peptides are the intended substrates for pancreatic enzymes, which complete the breakdown into amino acids. When unfolding is delayed or incomplete, larger protein fragments leave the stomach, requiring additional processing under conditions that are less optimal for initial structural change. This shifts the burden of transformation downstream and reduces overall efficiency.

Acid therefore functions as the gatekeeper of protein digestion by determining the physical accessibility of substrates. It does not simply contribute to digestion as one component among many. It defines whether the system can operate on proteins in a form that allows efficient enzymatic action. When this structural modification is fully established, the sequence proceeds with alignment between substrate and enzyme. When it is limited, the system is forced to process material that has not been properly prepared, and the effects extend through every subsequent stage.

Protein Unfolding and Enzymatic Access

Protein digestion depends on a change in structure that occurs before significant bond cleavage begins. In their native state, proteins are folded into compact configurations where many peptide bonds are buried within the interior of the molecule. These bonds are physically shielded by layers of secondary and tertiary structure, limiting direct contact with digestive enzymes. The stomach alters this arrangement through acid-driven unfolding, converting a tightly organized structure into an expanded form where internal regions become exposed. This shift is what determines whether enzymes can engage the substrate effectively.

As pH decreases in the gastric environment, the forces that stabilize protein folding are disrupted. Ionic interactions weaken as side chains gain or lose charge, hydrogen bonds are destabilized, and hydrophobic regions lose the structural context that keeps them sequestered. The protein transitions from a compact state into a more linear and flexible configuration. This change increases the number of accessible peptide bonds, allowing enzymes to attach and begin cleavage. Without this transition, enzyme activity is limited not by enzyme availability but by the inability to reach target sites.

Enzymatic access is governed by surface exposure. Proteolytic enzymes interact with specific sequences along the protein chain, but they can only act where those sequences are physically available. When unfolding is complete, the surface area of the protein increases, and previously hidden regions are presented for cleavage. This allows multiple enzymes to act simultaneously across different sites, accelerating the breakdown process. When unfolding is partial, access remains restricted, and enzymatic activity becomes uneven. Some regions are cleaved efficiently while others remain intact, resulting in a mixture of fragments that vary widely in size and structure.

The interaction between unfolding and enzyme activity also affects the rate and completeness of digestion. Early and sufficient unfolding allows enzymes to begin cleavage immediately upon activation, generating smaller peptides that are easier to process in subsequent stages. Delayed or incomplete unfolding slows this progression. Enzymes may still act on exposed regions, but the overall reduction of the protein is limited by the persistence of folded domains. These larger fragments move forward into the small intestine, where pancreatic enzymes must attempt to complete the process under conditions that are less effective for initial structural change.

This relationship between structure and access extends to the organization of food matrices. Proteins within connective tissue or complex food structures require both acid exposure and mechanical disruption to become accessible. When these processes are aligned, proteins are released from their surrounding matrix and unfolded in a way that allows enzymes to act uniformly. When alignment is lacking, portions of the protein remain embedded within intact structures, reducing the efficiency of enzymatic cleavage and increasing variability in the material that progresses through the system.

Protein unfolding and enzymatic access therefore form a single functional unit within digestion. The extent to which proteins are unfolded determines how effectively enzymes can perform their role. When structural modification is complete, enzymatic activity proceeds with high efficiency and consistency. When it is limited, enzyme function is constrained by physical barriers, and the sequence of digestion carries forward substrates that have not been adequately prepared for complete breakdown.

Acid Timing vs Acid Quantity

The effectiveness of gastric acid is determined less by how much is produced in total and more by when it is available relative to the arrival of food. Acid that is present at the moment food enters the stomach creates immediate conditions for protein unfolding and enzyme activation. Acid that is produced later must act on material that has already accumulated, altering the sequence of transformation and reducing the efficiency of early processing. The system depends on alignment between secretion and intake. When that alignment is present, digestion begins at full capacity. When it is delayed, the entire sequence starts from a lower baseline.

Early acid availability allows proteins to encounter a low pH environment as soon as they enter the stomach. Structural unfolding begins immediately, and proteolytic enzymes are activated in parallel. This synchrony ensures that mechanical mixing and chemical transformation occur together, producing a more uniform substrate for downstream processing. When acid production rises in advance or in real time with ingestion, the stomach operates as a prepared environment rather than a reactive one. Each incoming portion of food is processed under conditions that support consistent transformation.

Delayed acid production changes the dynamics of this process. Food enters a stomach that has not yet reached an effective pH, and proteins remain in a more intact state during the initial phase of mixing. The stomach attempts to increase acid output after detecting the presence of food, but this creates a lag between arrival and effective processing. During this period, material is exposed to mechanical forces without sufficient chemical alteration, leading to uneven breakdown. Some portions may begin to unfold as acid levels rise, while others remain structurally resistant. This variability carries forward into subsequent stages.

Total acid quantity can be adequate over the duration of digestion while still failing to produce optimal outcomes if timing is misaligned. A large volume of acid delivered late does not fully compensate for the absence of acid at the beginning. Early-stage transformations set the trajectory for the rest of the sequence, and once material has progressed without proper unfolding, downstream processes must compensate. Enzymes encounter substrates that have not been prepared, and the small intestine receives material that requires additional processing under less favorable conditions.

Timing also influences gastric emptying. When acid is available early, the stomach can regulate the release of its contents based on the degree of processing that has occurred. Material is retained until it has been sufficiently altered, and then released in a controlled manner. When acid is delayed, the stomach may either retain material longer to compensate or release it before complete processing has occurred. Both scenarios disrupt coordination with the small intestine, affecting enzyme activity and nutrient absorption.

The distinction between timing and quantity reframes how gastric function is evaluated. Adequate total acid production does not guarantee effective digestion if that acid is not present when it is needed. The sequence depends on early alignment between secretion and intake, where acid is available at the moment it can influence structure and enzyme activation. When this alignment is restored, the system operates with greater consistency and efficiency. When it is absent, increasing total output alone does not resolve the underlying misalignment, and the effects continue to propagate through the digestive sequence.

Chapter 6

Gastric Coordination and Timing

The stomach operates as a coordinated system that integrates secretion, mechanical force, and controlled release. These functions are not independent. They are synchronized through neural and local feedback so that chemical transformation, physical breakdown, and emptying occur in alignment. The outcome depends on timing. When secretion, mixing, and release are matched to the state of the meal, the stomach delivers a substrate that the small intestine can process efficiently. When timing is disrupted, the stomach either releases material that is not prepared or retains it under conditions that alter its structure in unintended ways.

Gastric secretion sets the chemical environment, but its effectiveness depends on how it is distributed. Muscular contractions mix incoming food with acid and enzymes, exposing surfaces and driving structural change. This mixing must occur while acid is present at sufficient levels to unfold proteins and activate enzymes. If secretion lags behind mechanical activity, the stomach churns material that has not yet been chemically prepared, producing uneven transformation. If mixing is insufficient relative to secretion, regions of the meal remain less exposed, and processing becomes inconsistent. Coordination between these elements determines whether the substrate becomes uniform or remains heterogeneous.

Motility patterns within the stomach regulate how material is processed over time. Contractions in the body of the stomach move contents toward the distal region, where more forceful activity reduces particle size and promotes further mixing. This mechanical progression is linked to the chemical state of the meal. As proteins are unfolded and partially cleaved, and as the physical structure of the meal changes, the stomach adjusts its contractions to maintain effective processing. When coordination is intact, mechanical force is applied to material

that is already undergoing chemical transformation, reinforcing the breakdown process.

Gastric emptying is controlled through feedback that reflects both the degree of processing and the readiness of the small intestine. The stomach releases its contents in portions, allowing the intestine to handle a manageable load. This release depends on signals that indicate how well the material has been transformed and whether downstream systems are prepared. When timing is aligned, partially digested material enters the intestine under conditions that support enzymatic completion and absorption. When timing is disrupted, the stomach may release material too early, before sufficient chemical and mechanical processing has occurred, or too late, altering the internal environment and changing the behavior of the meal.

The composition of the meal influences how this coordination is executed. Proteins, fats, and other components generate signals that adjust secretion and motility. Fat content, for example, slows emptying and increases the need for coordinated bile delivery downstream. Protein content influences acid production and enzyme activation. The stomach integrates these signals to adjust its timing so that each component is processed appropriately. When early-phase signaling is strong, these adjustments occur with precision. When it is weak, the stomach operates with reduced information, and coordination becomes less accurate.

Disruption of gastric timing often originates from upstream factors. Weak cephalic activation, rapid intake, and reduced parasympathetic tone lower the initial output and delay the alignment of secretion and motility. The stomach begins processing without having reached the conditions required for effective transformation. This delay propagates through mixing and emptying, producing a sequence where each step is slightly out of sync with the others. The result is increased variability in how material is processed and delivered to the intestine.

Restoring gastric coordination requires re-establishing alignment between these elements. When secretion rises in advance, mixing distributes acid and enzymes across a well-prepared substrate, and emptying is regulated based on actual processing rather than compensation. The stomach then functions as an integrated system that prepares material for the next stage with consistency. Timing becomes the organizing principle that links structure, function, and outcome, allowing the digestive sequence to proceed without the need for downstream correction.

Sequential Release into the Small Intestine

The stomach does not empty as a single event. It releases its contents in controlled pulses, each portion shaped by the degree of chemical and mechanical processing that has already occurred. This sequential delivery determines how effectively the small intestine can complete digestion and absorb nutrients. The intestine is not designed to receive the entire gastric load at once. It operates on a continuous but regulated flow, where each incoming fraction is matched to available enzymatic activity, bile presence, and absorptive capacity.

Each release from the stomach reflects a checkpoint in processing. Material that has been sufficiently mixed, acidified, and structurally altered is permitted to pass through the pyloric region, while less prepared portions are retained for further transformation. This creates a gradient within the stomach, where more processed contents move forward and less processed contents remain behind. The sequence depends on this internal sorting. When it functions properly, the intestine receives a substrate that is already partially reduced and chemically conditioned for rapid enzymatic completion.

The timing of these releases is coordinated with signals from the small intestine. As each portion arrives, receptors in the intestinal lining assess its composition and adjust downstream activity. Enzyme secretion is increased or modulated based on the presence of peptides and lipids, and bile delivery is coordinated to match fat content. This feedback also influences the rate of subsequent gastric emptying. If the intestine is processing efficiently, the stomach continues releasing material at a steady pace. If the load exceeds capacity, signals are sent to slow further release, allowing the intestine to regain alignment.

When sequential release is disrupted, this coordination breaks down. Rapid emptying delivers large volumes of inadequately processed material into the intestine, overwhelming enzymatic systems and diluting bile. The result is incomplete breakdown and reduced absorption efficiency. On the other end, delayed or irregular emptying can lead to prolonged retention in the stomach, altering the internal environment and changing how the meal is processed. In both cases, the intestine receives material that does not match its current capacity, forcing compensatory adjustments in motility and secretion.

The physical state of the meal influences how effectively this sequence operates. Uniformly processed contents move through the pyloric region in a predictable manner, allowing consistent delivery into the intestine. Heterogeneous mixtures, where some portions are well processed and others remain structurally intact, disrupt this flow. Larger or less prepared particles are retained while smaller fractions pass through, increasing variability in what the intestine receives over time. This variability affects enzyme efficiency and the stability of absorption.

Sequential release therefore links gastric processing to intestinal function. It ensures that each stage of digestion receives material in a form and quantity that can be handled effectively. When this process is aligned, the intestine operates on a steady stream of substrates that match its enzymatic and absorptive capacity. When it is misaligned, the intestine must compensate for irregular input, and the efficiency of the entire system declines.

Regulation of Gastric Emptying

Gastric emptying is governed by a feedback system that links the state of the stomach to the capacity of the small intestine. The pyloric region acts as a control point, allowing only portions of the gastric contents to pass once they meet specific physical and chemical conditions. This regulation is not fixed. It adjusts continuously based on how well the meal has been processed and how prepared the intestine is to receive it. The stomach releases material in a way that attempts to maintain alignment between upstream transformation and downstream capacity.

The physical properties of the gastric contents influence this control. Particle size determines whether material can pass through the pyloric opening. Larger, less processed fragments are retained until further mechanical and chemical reduction occurs. Smaller, more uniform particles are permitted to move forward. This creates an internal sorting mechanism where the degree of breakdown dictates progression. Mechanical activity and acid-driven structural change work together to reduce particle size and alter consistency, gradually shifting material into a state that can be released.

Chemical signals generated by the meal further refine this process. The presence of proteins, fats, and partially digested components in the small intestine feeds back to the stomach through neural and hormonal pathways. These signals adjust the tone of the pyloric region and the pattern of gastric contractions. When the intestine is actively processing incoming material, signals reduce the rate of further release, allowing time for enzymatic breakdown and absorption. When the intestine is ready to receive more, the stomach increases the frequency of release events. This dynamic control prevents overload and maintains a manageable flow.

Fat content exerts a strong influence on this regulation. Lipids require coordinated bile delivery and enzymatic activity in the intestine, and the system adjusts gastric emptying to match this requirement. The presence of fat slows release, extending the time available for emulsification and enzymatic action downstream. This delay is not a passive consequence of the meal but an active adjustment that aligns gastric output with intestinal processing capacity. When signaling is intact, this adjustment occurs with precision. When signaling is weak or mistimed, fat may enter the intestine without sufficient coordination, reducing the efficiency of breakdown and absorption.

Acid exposure within the stomach also contributes to emptying control. Adequate acidification alters the structure of the meal and influences how quickly material can be reduced to a form that passes through the pylorus. When acid is present early and in sufficient amounts, structural modification progresses in parallel with mechanical mixing, allowing controlled and consistent release. When acid is delayed or insufficient, larger and less altered fragments persist, prolonging retention or leading to irregular release patterns as the system attempts to compensate.

Neural input from the parasympathetic system integrates these factors into a coordinated response. Strong parasympathetic tone supports balanced secretion, effective motility, and responsive pyloric control. When this tone is reduced, coordination weakens. The stomach may release material too quickly due to reduced regulatory signaling or retain it longer without effective processing. In both cases, the alignment between stomach and intestine is disrupted, and the sequence becomes less predictable.

Regulation of gastric emptying therefore reflects the combined influence of structure, chemistry, and signaling. It determines how material transitions from gastric processing to intestinal digestion and whether that transition occurs under conditions that support efficient breakdown and absorption. When this regulation is intact, the stomach delivers a steady, controlled flow that matches intestinal capacity. When it is disrupted, the intestine receives material that is either premature or delayed, and the efficiency of the entire system declines.

Acid as a Gatekeeper

Gastric acid determines when material is ready to leave the stomach by defining the chemical state required for progression. It sets the threshold that proteins and other components must reach before the pyloric region permits release. This function is not abstract. Acid changes the structure of the meal, reduces particle integrity, and establishes the conditions that signal readiness for the next stage. When acid exposure is sufficient and occurs early, the stomach can move material forward in a controlled sequence. When it is limited or delayed, the gatekeeping function weakens, and the timing of release becomes inconsistent.

The gatekeeping role begins with structural transformation. As acid unfolds proteins and alters connective components within the meal, the physical resistance of the material decreases. This allows mechanical activity to reduce particle size more effectively, bringing the contents into a range that can pass through the pyloric opening. Without this structural change, larger fragments persist and are retained longer. The stomach must continue processing under conditions that may not be optimal, increasing variability in how and when material is eventually released.

Acid also establishes the chemical environment that signals readiness to downstream systems. As the stomach contents reach a certain level of acidification, feedback mechanisms adjust pyloric tone and coordinate the transition into the small intestine. This ensures that the material entering the intestine has undergone the necessary initial transformation. When acid levels are appropriate, release occurs in a pattern that matches intestinal capacity, allowing enzymes and bile to act on substrates that are already partially prepared.

When acid production is delayed, the gate opens under less controlled conditions. Material may begin to move forward before adequate structural modification has occurred, delivering substrates that are more difficult to process in the intestine. Alternatively, the stomach may retain contents longer in an attempt to compensate, but without sufficient acid, this extended retention does not produce the required transformation. In both cases, the alignment between gastric processing and intestinal capacity is disrupted.

The gatekeeping function also influences the consistency of delivery. With adequate acid, the stomach releases portions of a meal that have been processed to a similar degree, creating a steady flow of substrates into the intestine. When acid is insufficient, the contents remain heterogeneous, and the release becomes irregular. Smaller, more processed fractions may pass through while larger, less prepared fragments are retained. This variability affects how enzymes and bile interact with incoming material and contributes to fluctuations in digestive efficiency.

Acid as a gatekeeper therefore links structural transformation to controlled progression through the digestive sequence. It determines whether the stomach can deliver material that is ready for the next stage and whether that delivery occurs with consistent timing. When this function is intact, the transition into the small intestine is regulated and aligned with downstream capacity. When it is impaired, the sequence becomes disordered, and the effects extend through every subsequent stage of digestion.

PART IV

WHEN THE STOMACH FAILS

Chapter 7

Downstream Chaos

Downstream chaos emerges when early-stage constraints are carried forward into the small intestine, where precision is required but no longer possible. The intestine depends on receiving material that has been structurally modified, chemically conditioned, and delivered in controlled amounts. When those conditions are not met, the intestine does not fail in isolation. It attempts to compensate for upstream deficits using mechanisms that were not designed to handle poorly prepared substrates. The result is a system that remains active but loses coordination, where breakdown, absorption, motility, and microbial interaction begin to diverge from one another.

The first point of disruption appears in enzymatic breakdown. Pancreatic enzymes are calibrated to act on substrates that have already undergone partial reduction in the stomach. When larger, less processed proteins and fats arrive, enzyme efficiency decreases because access to cleavage sites is limited. Enzymes are present, but the structure of the material prevents consistent interaction. Some regions are reduced effectively while others persist, creating a mixture of fragments that vary in size and chemical composition. This variability is the starting point for downstream instability.

Bile coordination becomes less effective under these conditions. Lipids that have not been properly exposed or dispersed require more extensive emulsification, yet bile delivery depends on signaling that assumes a certain level of preparation. When this assumption is not met, bile may be insufficient relative to the state of the substrate. Fats remain in larger aggregates that resist enzymatic action, reducing the formation of transportable units. This alters not only fat absorption but also the physical environment within the intestine, influencing how other nutrients are processed.

Motility adjusts in response to these altered substrates. The intestine uses feedback from the lumen to regulate transit, attempting to balance exposure time with processing capacity. When breakdown is incomplete, the system may slow movement to increase contact time, or accelerate transit if irritation or osmotic effects are detected. These adjustments are reactive and often inconsistent. The timing between secretion, breakdown, and absorption loses alignment, and the sequence becomes less predictable from one segment of the intestine to the next.

Absorption efficiency declines as a direct consequence of these upstream and local disruptions. Nutrients that have not been reduced to their absorbable forms remain in the lumen, passing through transport regions without being taken up. The intestinal lining is presented with substrates that exceed its capacity to extract, leading to increased loss of usable material. At the same time, larger fragments and partially processed compounds continue moving distally, increasing the load on regions that are not optimized for primary digestion.

Microbial interaction intensifies as unprocessed material reaches the lower intestine. Substrates that would normally be absorbed earlier become available for fermentation, altering the composition and activity of microbial populations. This changes the chemical environment within the gut, producing compounds that can influence motility, barrier function, and immune signaling. These effects are not isolated to the microbial layer. They feed back into the host system, further increasing variability in digestion and absorption.

The system attempts to stabilize itself through compensation, but these compensations often introduce additional variability. Increased enzyme secretion, altered motility patterns, and shifts in fluid movement can partially offset the initial deficit, yet they do not restore alignment. Each adjustment is made in response to conditions that originated upstream, and the underlying sequence remains disrupted. The intestine continues to function, but it operates in a state where coordination between its components is reduced.

Downstream chaos is therefore the cumulative expression of early misalignment. It is not caused by a single failure within the intestine but by the propagation of constraints that began before the stomach completed its work. When early-phase signaling, acid timing, and gastric coordination are restored, the substrate entering the intestine changes. It arrives in a form that matches enzymatic and absorptive capacity, allowing the system to operate with consistency. Without that restoration, the intestine remains in a reactive state, continually adjusting to inputs that do not align with its design.

Sequential Failure Propagation

Digestion operates as a dependent chain where each stage inherits the output of the previous one, and any deficit introduced early is carried forward as a structural constraint rather than a transient error. When the initial phases begin below capacity, the system does not reset at the next stage. It builds on what it has been given. Weak sensory activation lowers early secretory output, delayed acid limits protein unfolding, and incomplete gastric processing delivers substrates that are not aligned with intestinal requirements. Each step receives material that is already compromised, and the sequence progresses with that constraint embedded in the system.

The propagation begins with altered substrate structure. Proteins that have not been fully unfolded retain regions that resist enzymatic access, and fats that have not been properly exposed remain in aggregates that limit emulsification. These structural features are not corrected automatically downstream. Pancreatic enzymes act on what is available, but their efficiency is governed by access to specific sites. When access is restricted, breakdown becomes uneven. Some components are reduced while others persist, creating a heterogeneous mixture that continues through the intestine with varying levels of preparation.

This heterogeneity drives secondary adjustments in secretion and motility. The intestine attempts to match its output to the state of the material it receives, increasing enzyme release where possible and altering transit speed to extend or reduce exposure time. These adjustments are local responses to upstream conditions. They do not restore the original sequence but attempt to compensate within a system that is already misaligned. The result is a pattern where different segments of the intestine operate under different conditions, each responding to the same substrate in its own way.

As partially processed material moves further along, the burden shifts to regions that are not designed for primary digestion. Larger fragments and unabsorbed nutrients reach distal sections of the gut, where microbial populations interact with them. This introduces additional variables into the system, including changes in luminal composition and chemical signaling. These changes feed back into motility and secretion, further altering the behavior of the digestive tract. The sequence becomes increasingly complex, with multiple layers of response acting on a substrate that was never properly prepared.

The key feature of this propagation is that each stage amplifies the effects of the previous one. A small deficit in early signaling can lead to a larger disruption in gastric processing, which then produces a more significant mismatch in the intestine. The system does not fail at a single point. It accumulates deviations from alignment, and those deviations interact with one another. By the time material reaches the distal gut, the original cause is no longer visible as a single event, but its effects are embedded in the behavior of the entire sequence.

Reversing this pattern requires intervention at the level where the sequence begins. Strengthening early signaling, restoring acid timing, and aligning gastric coordination change the structure of the substrate before it enters the intestine. When the initial output is corrected, each downstream stage receives material that matches its design parameters, and the need for compensation decreases. The sequence regains continuity because each step is now building on a properly prepared input rather than attempting to correct an inherited deficit.

Compensation Across the Intestine

When the intestine receives material that has not been properly prepared upstream, it does not stop functioning. It shifts its behavior in an attempt to manage the load, adjusting secretion, motility, and absorption in ways that partially offset the deficit. These compensations are driven by local sensing of luminal contents and are applied segment by segment. The intestine is not correcting the original problem. It is redistributing effort across its length to maintain forward movement and extract what it can from a substrate that exceeds its designed processing conditions.

Enzymatic compensation is the first response. Pancreatic output can increase in response to the presence of larger or more complex substrates, raising the concentration of digestive enzymes in the lumen. This increase improves breakdown where access is available, but it does not change the underlying structure of resistant regions. Enzymes act where they can reach, leaving portions of the substrate only partially reduced. The result is a mixture that still contains fragments too large or too complex for efficient absorption, even though enzyme activity has been elevated.

Motility adjusts in parallel. The intestine modulates transit speed based on the chemical and physical characteristics of the contents it detects. When breakdown is incomplete, transit may slow to extend exposure time, allowing enzymes more opportunity to act and absorption mechanisms more time to engage. In other situations, particularly when unprocessed material alters osmotic balance or irritates the lining, transit may accelerate. These opposing adjustments reflect an attempt to stabilize the system under variable conditions. The sequence becomes less predictable because transit is no longer governed by a consistent processing timeline.

Fluid movement is also altered as part of this compensation. The intestine regulates secretion and reabsorption of water to maintain a workable environment for enzymatic activity and nutrient transport. When substrates remain in larger or more complex forms, fluid dynamics can shift to facilitate dispersion or to manage osmotic gradients. These changes influence the consistency of the luminal contents and affect how enzymes and bile interact with the substrate. Variability in fluid handling contributes to fluctuations in how efficiently nutrients are extracted.

Absorptive mechanisms operate under these altered conditions with reduced efficiency. Transport systems in the intestinal lining are optimized for specific molecular forms. When substrates have not been fully reduced, these transporters are underutilized because the required forms are not present in sufficient quantities. The intestine may increase surface interaction through changes in motility and contact time, but the limitation remains structural. Larger fragments continue moving forward, carrying potential energy that is not being captured.

As these compensations occur, the distribution of workload across the intestine shifts. Proximal regions attempt to handle a greater burden, while distal regions receive material that would normally have been absorbed earlier. This redistribution introduces new interactions, particularly with microbial populations that encounter substrates in forms and quantities that differ from baseline conditions. The chemical environment of the lumen changes, and these changes feed back into motility, secretion, and barrier function.

Compensation across the intestine therefore reflects a system attempting to maintain function without restoring alignment. Each adjustment addresses an immediate constraint but introduces variability that affects subsequent stages. The intestine continues to process and absorb, but it does so under conditions that are less stable and less efficient. The underlying sequence remains disrupted because the initial preparation of the substrate has not been corrected, and every compensatory action is layered onto that original constraint.

Motility Disruption and Unpredictability

Intestinal motility is organized to move material forward while maintaining alignment between secretion, breakdown, and absorption. This coordination depends on receiving substrates that have been processed to a predictable state. When upstream transformation is incomplete, the signals that govern motility become inconsistent because they are derived from a substrate that varies in structure and composition. The intestine adjusts its movement based on what it detects in the lumen, and when that input is unstable, the resulting motility patterns lose coherence.

Segmental contractions and propulsive waves are normally timed to allow enzymes to act and nutrients to be absorbed before material advances. When partially processed substrates enter the intestine, this timing is altered. Larger fragments and unevenly reduced components trigger local responses that either slow movement to increase exposure or accelerate it when the system detects conditions that require rapid clearance. These opposing adjustments can occur within the same region over short intervals, producing a pattern that shifts between retention and rapid transit. The sequence no longer follows a consistent rhythm.

Chemical signaling contributes to this variability. The presence of unprocessed proteins, lipids, and other compounds influences the release of mediators that regulate smooth muscle activity. When substrates are not in their expected forms, these signals do not align with the standard progression of digestion. Motility is driven by inputs that fluctuate in both intensity and timing, leading to contractions that are not synchronized with enzymatic activity or absorptive capacity. The intestine continues to move contents forward, but the relationship between movement and processing becomes unstable.

Fluid dynamics further interact with these changes. Variations in osmotic load and luminal composition influence how water is secreted or absorbed, altering the consistency of the contents. Changes in consistency affect how easily material can be propelled and how it interacts with the intestinal wall. Thinner contents may move more rapidly, while thicker or more heterogeneous mixtures may be retained longer. These physical differences feed back into motility patterns, adding another layer of variability to an already unstable system.

The cumulative effect is unpredictability in transit time and processing efficiency. Material may pass through sections of the intestine too quickly for complete enzymatic breakdown and absorption, or it may remain longer in other sections without achieving the necessary transformation. The system oscillates between states rather than maintaining a stable progression. Each adjustment is a response to local conditions, but those conditions are shaped by upstream deficits that have not been resolved.

Motility disruption therefore reflects a loss of coordinated timing across the digestive sequence. It is not a failure of movement itself but a breakdown in how movement is regulated relative to processing and absorption. When upstream alignment is restored, the signals that govern motility become more consistent, and the intestine returns to a pattern where propulsion and processing are synchronized. Without that alignment, motility remains reactive, and the sequence continues to operate with variability that cannot be stabilized at the level of movement alone.

Microbial Shifts and Fermentation

The composition and activity of microbial populations in the intestine are determined by the substrates that reach them. When upstream digestion is aligned, most proteins, fats, and simple carbohydrates are reduced and absorbed before they can serve as fuel for microbial metabolism in distal regions. When early processing is incomplete, larger fragments and unabsorbed nutrients move forward, altering the substrate field that microbes encounter. This shift changes which populations expand, how they metabolize available material, and what byproducts are produced within the lumen.

Fermentation increases when substrates that should have been absorbed earlier remain available. Microbes break down these compounds into smaller molecules, generating gases and organic acids that alter the chemical environment. The rate and pattern of fermentation depend on the type of substrate present. Partially digested proteins, residual carbohydrates, and unprocessed fats each support different metabolic pathways within the microbial community. As these pathways become more active, the balance between microbial groups shifts toward those that can utilize the available material most efficiently.

These changes influence the physical state of the intestine. Gas production affects luminal pressure and can alter motility patterns, while organic acids modify pH and influence the activity of both microbes and host enzymes. The intestinal lining is exposed to compounds that vary depending on the substrates being fermented, and these compounds can affect barrier function and signaling pathways that regulate immune and neural responses. The system responds to these changes, but the responses are shaped by the altered environment rather than by the original design of the digestive sequence.

The timing of substrate delivery also affects microbial behavior. When gastric emptying and intestinal motility are inconsistent, substrates arrive in irregular pulses rather than in a steady flow. Microbial populations respond to these fluctuations, expanding when substrate is abundant and contracting when it is limited. This variability contributes to instability in the microbial ecosystem, where shifts in population dynamics can occur over relatively short periods. The chemical outputs of these populations then fluctuate in parallel, influencing motility, secretion, and absorption.

Microbial shifts therefore represent a downstream expression of upstream inefficiency. The intestine is not only processing nutrients for the host but also managing a secondary system that responds to what remains unabsorbed. When digestion is aligned, microbial activity is supported by a controlled and limited substrate supply that maintains stability. When digestion is disrupted, excess and inconsistent substrates drive changes in microbial composition and metabolic output, introducing additional variability into the system.

These changes feed back into the host, affecting how the intestine regulates movement, fluid balance, and barrier integrity. The system adapts to the altered microbial environment, but these adaptations are layered onto the original disruption. The result is a digestive sequence that is influenced not only by incomplete upstream processing but also by the secondary effects of microbial metabolism acting on substrates that should not have reached that stage in their original form.

Immune Activation from Incomplete Digestion

The intestinal immune system is positioned to respond to material that reaches the epithelial surface, and its level of activation depends on how completely that material has been reduced before arrival. When digestion proceeds with proper sequencing, proteins are broken down into small peptides and amino acids that can be transported across the epithelial layer with minimal interaction with immune surveillance systems. When upstream processing is incomplete, larger fragments persist within the lumen and come into contact with the mucosal interface. These fragments present structural features that are more likely to be recognized as signals requiring attention, increasing the likelihood of immune activation.

The barrier between the lumen and the internal environment is selective, relying on both physical structure and transport mechanisms to regulate what passes through. When substrates are in their intended forms, they are absorbed through controlled pathways that limit exposure to immune cells. Larger, partially digested fragments do not follow these pathways efficiently. They may remain in the lumen, interacting with the epithelial surface, or they may cross in ways that engage immune detection systems. This interaction is not random. It is driven by the structural properties of the material that has not been fully reduced.

Local immune responses are triggered when these interactions reach a threshold. Cells within the intestinal lining detect patterns associated with incomplete digestion and respond by releasing signaling molecules that influence both immune activity and epithelial behavior. This can alter barrier function, change fluid dynamics, and affect motility. The response is designed to manage potential threats, but when the stimulus is persistent, the system remains in a state of ongoing activation. This shifts the baseline condition of the intestine, affecting how it processes subsequent meals.

The presence of partially digested material also interacts with microbial activity, amplifying immune signaling. Microbial populations metabolize these substrates, producing compounds that can further influence the epithelial environment. These compounds may enhance or prolong immune responses, creating a feedback loop where incomplete digestion and microbial metabolism reinforce one another. The immune system responds to both the original substrate and the products of microbial processing, increasing the overall level of activation within the gut.

This activation has functional consequences for digestion. Changes in barrier behavior can influence absorption, while alterations in motility can affect transit time and the distribution of substrates along the intestine. Fluid movement may be adjusted in response to immune signaling, modifying the consistency of luminal contents. These changes are not isolated effects. They are part of a coordinated response that attempts to manage the presence of material that has not been properly processed upstream.

Immune activation in this context reflects a mismatch between substrate and system capacity. The intestine is encountering forms of material that it is not designed to handle under normal conditions, and it responds accordingly. When upstream digestion is restored, the nature of the material reaching the intestinal surface changes. Smaller, fully reduced substrates interact with the epithelium through established transport pathways, reducing the need for immune engagement. The system returns to a state where immune activity is aligned with actual threats rather than with the byproducts of incomplete digestion.

System-Wide Symptoms from Upstream Failure

When digestion begins below capacity, the effects are not confined to the gut. The digestive sequence supplies substrates, signals, and regulatory inputs to multiple systems, and when that sequence is disrupted early, the outputs that reach the rest of the body are altered in both quantity and form. Incomplete protein breakdown limits the availability of amino acids required for tissue maintenance, enzyme production, and signaling pathways. Impaired fat processing reduces the delivery of lipid components that support membrane structure and signaling. These changes shift the internal environment, and the body responds with adjustments that are experienced as symptoms across different systems.

Energy regulation is one of the first areas affected. Nutrient absorption becomes inconsistent when substrates are not fully reduced, leading to fluctuations in the availability of usable fuel. The body attempts to stabilize this variability through hormonal adjustments that alter how energy is stored and released. These adjustments can produce patterns of fatigue, unstable energy levels, and changes in appetite. The underlying driver is not a lack of intake but a mismatch between intake and the system's ability to convert that intake into accessible substrates.

The immune system reflects these changes as well. Increased exposure to partially digested material and the byproducts of altered microbial activity raises baseline immune activation within the gut. Signals generated at the intestinal level extend beyond the local environment, influencing systemic immune behavior. This can manifest as a persistent state of low-level activation that affects how the body responds to additional challenges. The source of this activation is rooted in the material reaching the intestinal interface rather than in an external input alone.

Neurological signaling is also influenced by the state of digestion. The gut communicates with the central nervous system through neural and chemical pathways that respond to the condition of the digestive process. When digestion is inconsistent, these signals become less stable, affecting patterns of focus, mood, and perception of stress. The system interprets variability in nutrient delivery and immune signaling as changes in internal conditions, and neural output adjusts accordingly. This creates a link between digestive function and cognitive or emotional states.

Fluid balance and circulation can shift as the body responds to altered digestive conditions. Changes in intestinal permeability, motility, and secretion influence how fluids are distributed and retained. These shifts can affect tissue hydration, circulation patterns, and the delivery of nutrients to peripheral systems. The body compensates for these changes, but the compensation reflects the underlying disruption rather than correcting it.

Symptom clustering often emerges from this pattern of system-wide adjustment. Fatigue, digestive discomfort, variability in energy, and changes in immune or neurological function appear together because they share a common origin in upstream digestive failure. Each system is responding to the same set of altered inputs, and the overlap in symptoms reflects the interconnected nature of these responses.

Restoring upstream function changes the inputs that drive these system-wide effects. When digestion proceeds with proper sequencing, nutrients are delivered in their intended forms, immune activation is reduced, and signaling between systems stabilizes. The body no longer needs to compensate for inconsistent inputs, and the pattern of symptoms begins to resolve as the underlying sequence is brought back into alignment.

Chapter 8

Delayed Gastric Emptying

Delayed gastric emptying reflects a breakdown in the coordination between chemical transformation, mechanical processing, and controlled release. The stomach is designed to hold material until it has been sufficiently altered, then deliver it forward in measured portions that match intestinal capacity. When this timing is extended beyond what is required for proper processing, the internal environment of the stomach changes, and the sequence begins to diverge from its intended pattern. The delay is not simply a matter of slower movement. It is a shift in how long material remains under conditions that were meant to be transitional rather than prolonged.

The initial driver of delayed emptying is often a mismatch between acid availability and substrate load. When acid production is insufficient or delayed, proteins are not unfolded efficiently, and the structural reduction required for progression is incomplete. The stomach retains material in an attempt to continue processing, but without adequate acid, this extended retention does not achieve the necessary transformation. Mechanical activity continues, but it operates on a substrate that remains resistant, leading to a state where time is increased without a proportional increase in processing quality.

Motility patterns adapt to this condition by reducing the rate of forward propulsion. The pyloric region remains more closed, and the release of material into the small intestine slows. This adjustment is driven by feedback that indicates the substrate is not ready for progression. At the same time, contractions within the stomach may become less coordinated, as the system attempts to balance mixing with retention.

The result is a pattern where material is held longer while being exposed to mechanical forces that do not fully resolve the underlying structural constraints.

As retention increases, the internal environment of the stomach shifts. Prolonged exposure to partially processed material alters the chemical and physical state of the contents. Components of the meal that would normally move forward begin to interact within the stomach for extended periods, changing how they behave when eventually released. This can affect the consistency of the material and the pattern of release, leading to less predictable delivery into the small intestine.

Downstream effects emerge as the intestine receives material in a delayed and often uneven manner. The timing of enzyme secretion and bile delivery is based on signals that assume a certain progression of gastric emptying. When this progression is altered, coordination is reduced. The intestine may receive smaller, intermittent releases followed by larger pulses, disrupting the alignment between substrate arrival and processing capacity. This variability affects enzymatic efficiency and absorption, contributing to instability in the digestive sequence.

Neural regulation plays a central role in this process. Reduced parasympathetic tone lowers both secretory output and coordinated motility, creating conditions where the stomach retains material without effectively processing it. The system remains active, but its components are no longer synchronized. The delay becomes a compensatory state that reflects upstream deficits rather than an isolated dysfunction of movement.

Delayed gastric emptying therefore represents a persistence of material within the stomach that exceeds the time required for proper transformation under aligned conditions. It is the result of insufficient preparation combined with altered coordination, where the system attempts to correct a deficit by extending retention. Without restoring the underlying factors that drive effective processing and timing, this extended retention continues to alter the sequence, affecting both the stomach and the stages that follow.

Failed Preparation Leading to Retention

Retention in the stomach is often the direct consequence of incomplete preparation rather than a primary failure of movement. The stomach holds material when the conditions required for progression have not been met. Acid exposure has not sufficiently altered protein structure, particle size remains too large, and the chemical signals that indicate readiness for release are weak or inconsistent. Under these conditions, the pyloric region limits forward flow because the substrate does not match the requirements of the small intestine. The system is not arbitrarily delaying emptying. It is preventing the transfer of material that would be difficult to process downstream.

This failure begins before the stomach has fully engaged. Weak cephalic activation reduces early acid output, and rapid intake limits both mechanical breakdown and anticipatory signaling. Food enters the stomach without having triggered the level of secretion required for immediate transformation. The stomach responds by increasing acid production after the fact, but this creates a lag where material is present without the chemical environment needed to alter it. During this period, mechanical mixing occurs on a substrate that remains structurally resistant, leading to uneven and incomplete preparation.

As this condition persists, the stomach shifts into a retention mode. Contractions continue to mix contents, but forward propulsion is reduced because the signals that would normally permit release are not being generated. Larger and less processed fragments are held back, while only smaller portions may pass intermittently. This selective retention reflects an attempt to continue processing until the substrate reaches a state that can move forward. Without sufficient acid or proper timing, this extended processing does not fully resolve the structural limitations, and retention continues.

The internal environment changes as material remains in the stomach longer than intended. Components of the meal interact under conditions that were designed to be transient, altering the consistency and behavior of the contents. The longer material is retained without adequate transformation, the more heterogeneous the mixture becomes. When release eventually occurs, it often does so in irregular patterns, sending unevenly processed material into the small intestine.

Downstream coordination is affected by this irregular delivery. The intestine receives material that arrives later than expected and in forms that do not match its enzymatic capacity. Signals that regulate enzyme secretion and bile flow are based on timing that assumes proper gastric progression. When this timing is altered, these processes lose alignment. The intestine attempts to compensate, but the substrate it receives has already been shaped by prolonged and incomplete gastric processing.

Failed preparation leading to retention therefore reflects a breakdown in the conditions required for progression rather than an isolated delay in movement. The stomach is holding material because it has not been adequately transformed, and without restoring the factors that enable that transformation, retention persists as a compensatory state. The sequence remains disrupted because the initial deficit has not been corrected, and each stage continues to operate on a substrate that does not meet its requirements.

Protective Slowing Mechanisms

Slowing within the digestive system is not inherently pathological. It is often a protective response that emerges when the substrate entering the intestine does not match the system's capacity to process it. The stomach and small intestine adjust the rate of movement to prevent overload, limit exposure to poorly prepared material, and preserve the integrity of downstream processing. This slowing is driven by feedback that detects the chemical and physical state of the contents, and it acts to maintain control over a sequence that would otherwise become unstable.

The first layer of this protection occurs at the level of gastric emptying. When the stomach detects that proteins have not been sufficiently unfolded or that fats have not been properly prepared for emulsification, signals reduce the rate of release into the small intestine. The pyloric region maintains a higher level of closure, allowing only small amounts of material to pass at a time. This reduces the immediate burden on the intestine and creates additional time for ongoing gastric processing. The stomach is attempting to improve the condition of the substrate before allowing it to move forward.

Within the small intestine, slowing continues as a secondary response. When partially processed material arrives, local sensing mechanisms detect the mismatch between substrate structure and enzymatic capacity. In response, motility patterns shift to increase contact time between the contents and the intestinal lining. This extended exposure allows enzymes more opportunity to act and gives absorption mechanisms additional time to extract available nutrients. The system is compensating for reduced efficiency by increasing duration.

Chemical signals play a central role in coordinating this slowing. The presence of fats, larger peptides, and other incompletely processed components triggers the release of mediators that influence both gastric and intestinal motility. These signals reduce forward propulsion and adjust the timing of subsequent releases from the stomach. The effect is a coordinated reduction in speed that spans multiple segments of the digestive tract. When signaling is aligned, this slowing is precise and proportional to the state of the substrate.

However, when upstream preparation remains inadequate, protective slowing can become prolonged and less effective. Extended retention in the stomach does not resolve structural resistance if acid levels are insufficient, and prolonged contact time in the intestine does not fully compensate for limited enzymatic access. The system continues to slow movement in an attempt to regain alignment, but the underlying conditions remain unchanged. This leads to a state where time is increased without a corresponding improvement in processing quality.

The consequence of sustained slowing is a shift in the internal environment. Material remains in contact with the intestinal lining for longer periods, and microbial interactions become more pronounced as substrates persist within the lumen. These changes introduce additional variables into the system, influencing motility, secretion, and absorption in ways that further complicate the sequence. The protective mechanism begins to contribute to variability rather than stability.

Protective slowing mechanisms therefore represent an adaptive response to upstream failure. They are designed to preserve function by reducing the rate at which the system is challenged, but they do not correct the initial deficit. When early-stage preparation is restored, the need for slowing diminishes, and the system returns to a pattern where timing is governed by coordinated processing rather than by compensation.

Fermentation and Pressure Buildup

When material remains in the digestive tract longer than intended or reaches distal regions without adequate processing, microbial fermentation increases and changes the physical state of the lumen. Substrates that would normally be reduced and absorbed earlier become available to microbial populations, which metabolize them into gases and smaller chemical compounds. This process is not inherently disruptive, but when it is driven by excess or poorly prepared material, the rate and volume of gas production increase beyond what the system can easily manage. The result is a rise in luminal pressure that affects both motility and the perception of discomfort.

Gas accumulation alters the mechanical environment of the intestine. As pressure builds, the intestinal wall stretches, activating sensory pathways that signal distension. This distension can modify motility patterns, either slowing movement to reduce further accumulation or triggering irregular contractions that attempt to redistribute or expel the contents. These adjustments are reactive and depend on the local conditions within each segment. The coordination between propulsion and processing is reduced because movement is now influenced by pressure rather than by the normal sequencing of digestion.

The distribution of gas within the intestine also affects how contents are mixed and transported. Pockets of gas can separate regions of the luminal contents, creating areas where enzymatic contact is reduced. This further limits the breakdown of substrates that are already incompletely processed. At the same time, pressure gradients can shift the movement of fluids, altering the consistency of the contents and influencing how easily they can be propelled. These changes add variability to a system that is already operating under constrained conditions.

Chemical byproducts of fermentation contribute to this environment. Organic acids and other compounds produced by microbial metabolism modify the pH and interact with the intestinal lining. These changes can influence both motility and secretion, reinforcing the effects of mechanical pressure. The intestine responds to these signals, but the responses are shaped by the altered conditions rather than by the original design of the digestive sequence.

As pressure builds and motility adjusts, the timing of movement becomes less predictable. Material may be retained in certain regions while moving more rapidly through others, creating a pattern where processing and propulsion are no longer synchronized. This variability affects absorption, as some substrates may not remain in contact with the intestinal lining long enough to be fully taken up, while others are exposed for extended periods without achieving complete breakdown.

Fermentation and pressure buildup therefore represent a downstream consequence of incomplete upstream processing combined with altered transit. The increase in microbial activity and gas production changes the mechanical and chemical environment of the intestine, influencing how material moves and how effectively it is processed. Without restoring the conditions that limit excess substrate delivery to these regions, pressure and its associated effects continue to shape the behavior of the system.

Transition Failure Between Stomach and Intestine

The junction between the stomach and small intestine is a controlled handoff where material that has been chemically and mechanically prepared is delivered into an environment designed to complete digestion and initiate absorption. This transition depends on alignment between what the stomach produces and what the intestine is ready to receive. When that alignment is lost, the interface becomes a point of failure rather than a point of continuity. The intestine receives material that does not match its operating conditions, and the sequence shifts from coordinated progression to reactive adjustment.

The stomach is responsible for delivering a substrate that has undergone sufficient acid exposure and mechanical reduction. This preparation determines whether enzymes in the small intestine can access and complete the breakdown of macromolecules. When proteins are not fully unfolded or when fats remain in larger aggregates, the material entering the intestine carries structural resistance. The intestine is equipped to finish digestion, but it is not designed to initiate the level of transformation that should have occurred upstream. The mismatch begins at the moment of entry.

Timing is central to this transition. Gastric emptying is normally synchronized with intestinal signaling so that enzyme secretion and bile delivery are aligned with the arrival of partially processed material. When this timing is disrupted, the intestine receives material either too early, before adequate preparation has occurred, or too late, after prolonged retention has altered its structure. In both cases, coordination between stages is reduced. Enzymes may be present without appropriate substrates, or substrates may arrive without sufficient enzymatic or biliary support.

The chemical environment at the interface also depends on this alignment. Material leaving the stomach carries the conditions created by gastric processing, including its degree of acidification. The small intestine adjusts its own environment in response to this incoming material, regulating pH and enzyme activity accordingly. When the composition of the gastric output is inconsistent, these adjustments become less precise. The intestine must respond to a variable input, and the stability of its internal conditions is reduced.

Motility at this junction reflects the same dependency. The controlled release of gastric contents is designed to match intestinal capacity, allowing for steady progression. When release becomes irregular, the intestine experiences fluctuations in load. Smaller amounts may be followed by larger pulses, disrupting the timing of enzymatic activity and absorption. The system compensates by altering transit speed and secretion patterns, but these compensations do not restore the original coordination.

The consequences of transition failure extend through the remainder of the digestive tract. Substrates that are not properly matched to intestinal capacity continue forward in partially processed forms, influencing microbial activity, immune signaling, and nutrient absorption. Each downstream stage inherits the effects of the initial mismatch, and variability increases as the sequence progresses.

Transition failure between the stomach and intestine therefore represents a breakdown in the continuity of the digestive sequence. It is not a problem confined to either organ but a failure of coordination between them. Restoring this transition requires aligning gastric preparation with intestinal readiness so that material is delivered in a form and at a time that allows each stage to operate within its designed parameters.

PART V

THE SMALL INTESTINE AS A PROCESSING SYSTEM

Chapter 9

Enzymes and Breakdown

Enzymes drive the chemical reduction of food into absorbable units, but their effectiveness depends on the structural state of the substrate they encounter. They do not initiate digestion in isolation. They act on material that has already been altered by mechanical breakdown and gastric acid. The intestine is equipped with a broad array of enzymes capable of cleaving proteins, fats, and carbohydrates, yet these enzymes require access to specific sites within each molecule. When the substrate arrives in a form that exposes those sites, breakdown proceeds with high efficiency. When it does not, enzyme activity becomes limited by physical constraints rather than by enzyme availability.

Proteolytic enzymes in the small intestine complete the reduction of proteins into smaller peptides and amino acids. These enzymes are designed to act on substrates that have already been unfolded and partially cleaved in the stomach. When this preparation is adequate, the remaining peptide bonds are accessible, and enzymatic action proceeds in a coordinated manner. When upstream unfolding is incomplete, large segments of protein remain structurally resistant. Enzymes engage only the exposed regions, leaving intact domains that pass further along the intestine. The result is incomplete reduction and reduced availability of absorbable amino acids.

Lipolytic enzymes operate under a similar dependency. Fat digestion requires that lipids be dispersed into smaller units that can be accessed by enzymes. Bile plays a central role in this process by organizing fats into structures that increase surface area. When fats arrive in a properly prepared state, lipases can act efficiently, reducing triglycerides into components that can be absorbed. When fats remain in larger aggregates due to inadequate preparation, enzyme access is limited. Breakdown slows, and portions of dietary fat continue through the intestine without being fully processed.

Carbohydrate digestion also reflects this relationship between structure and enzymatic access. Enzymes act on specific linkages within carbohydrate molecules, and their activity depends on the availability of these linkages. When carbohydrates are presented in forms that allow enzyme contact, breakdown proceeds rapidly. When structural barriers persist, enzymatic action becomes uneven, producing a mixture of fully reduced and partially processed fragments. These fragments influence both absorption and microbial activity as they move through the intestine.

Enzyme secretion is regulated by signals that reflect the presence and composition of incoming material. The pancreas adjusts its output based on what is detected in the intestine, increasing enzyme delivery when demand is higher. This regulation assumes that substrates are within a range that enzymes can effectively process. When substrates fall outside that range due to upstream deficits, increased enzyme output cannot fully compensate. The limitation remains structural, and the efficiency of breakdown is constrained regardless of enzyme concentration.

The timing of enzyme activity is also critical. Enzymes must be present when substrates arrive in a state that allows interaction. When gastric emptying is irregular or when early-phase signaling is weak, the alignment between enzyme release and substrate availability is disrupted. Enzymes may be released into the intestine before or after the optimal window for interaction, reducing overall efficiency. This misalignment contributes to variability in how completely different portions of a meal are processed.

Enzymes and breakdown therefore function within the context of the entire digestive sequence. Their ability to reduce food into absorbable units depends on the preparation that occurs upstream and the timing of their release relative to substrate arrival. When the sequence is aligned, enzymes operate on substrates that are accessible and appropriately timed, producing consistent and efficient breakdown. When the sequence is disrupted, enzymatic activity is constrained by structural and temporal factors, and the products of digestion reflect that limitation.

Pancreatic Enzyme Dependency on Upstream Signals

Pancreatic enzyme output is not constant. It is scaled and timed according to signals that originate before and during the transition from stomach to small intestine. These signals inform the pancreas about the volume and composition of the meal and determine how much enzyme is released and when that release occurs. The system assumes that upstream processes have prepared the substrate to a predictable state. When those signals are accurate and timely, enzyme delivery aligns with substrate arrival. When they are weak or mistimed, pancreatic output becomes mismatched to the material entering the intestine.

Early signaling begins before food reaches the small intestine. Sensory input and gastric activity generate neural signals that prime pancreatic secretion. This preparatory phase raises baseline output so that enzymes are available as soon as partially processed material begins to enter the duodenum. As gastric contents move forward, additional signals are generated based on the chemical composition of the incoming material. These signals further adjust enzyme release, increasing output when proteins, fats, or carbohydrates are present in forms that require breakdown.

The effectiveness of this system depends on the integrity of upstream processing. When proteins have been unfolded and partially cleaved in the stomach, and when fats have been exposed and dispersed, the signals generated at the intestinal level accurately reflect the state of the substrate. The pancreas responds by delivering enzymes that can immediately act on accessible targets. Breakdown proceeds with coordination between substrate and enzyme, and the sequence advances efficiently.

When upstream processing is incomplete, the signals that drive pancreatic output become less reliable. Larger, less processed substrates may not trigger the same level of response, or they may generate signals that do not correspond to the actual difficulty of breakdown. The pancreas may release enzymes in amounts that are insufficient relative to the structural resistance of the material, or the timing of release may not align with substrate arrival. In these conditions, enzymes are present but cannot fully engage with the substrate, and the efficiency of digestion declines.

Timing is a critical component of this dependency. Enzymes must be delivered into the intestine at the moment when substrates are available and accessible. When gastric emptying is irregular or when early-phase signaling is reduced, this alignment is disrupted. Enzymes may be released too early, before substrates arrive, or too late, after portions of the substrate have already moved beyond the optimal region for interaction. This temporal mismatch reduces the effectiveness of enzymatic breakdown even when total enzyme output is adequate.

The system attempts to compensate for these mismatches by adjusting enzyme secretion based on ongoing feedback, but this compensation is limited by the structural state of the substrate. Increasing enzyme concentration does not overcome restricted access to cleavage sites within intact or poorly prepared molecules. The limitation remains at the level of substrate preparation, and the pancreas continues to operate within constraints that it cannot resolve independently.

Pancreatic enzyme dependency on upstream signals therefore reflects the integrated nature of digestion. The pancreas relies on accurate and timely information from earlier stages to align its output with the needs of the system. When upstream processes are functioning properly, this alignment allows enzymes to operate at full efficiency. When they are not, pancreatic output becomes misaligned with substrate conditions, and the breakdown of food proceeds with reduced consistency and effectiveness.

Protein, Fat, and Carbohydrate Processing

The breakdown of proteins, fats, and carbohydrates follows a coordinated sequence in which each macronutrient is transformed according to its structure and the conditions established upstream. These processes do not operate independently. They are linked through shared requirements for timing, substrate preparation, and signaling. The efficiency of each pathway depends on whether the material entering the small intestine has been properly altered in the stomach and whether enzyme delivery and bile coordination align with that material.

Protein processing begins with acid-driven unfolding in the stomach, which exposes peptide bonds and allows proteolytic enzymes to initiate cleavage. By the time proteins reach the small intestine, they are expected to be in the form of smaller peptides. Pancreatic enzymes then complete the reduction into amino acids and short peptide fragments that can be transported across the intestinal lining. When this sequence is aligned, protein breakdown proceeds with high efficiency because enzymes are acting on substrates that are structurally accessible. When unfolding and early cleavage are incomplete, larger protein fragments persist, limiting enzymatic access and reducing the availability of absorbable amino acids.

Fat processing depends on both structural dispersion and coordinated bile delivery. Lipids must be broken into smaller units that can be acted on by lipolytic enzymes. Bile organizes fats into structures that increase surface area, allowing enzymes to access and cleave them into absorbable components. This process requires that fats arrive in a state that can be effectively emulsified. When upstream preparation exposes lipids adequately and signaling aligns bile release with substrate arrival, breakdown proceeds efficiently. When fats remain in larger aggregates or bile delivery is mistimed, enzymatic access is reduced, and portions of dietary fat move through the intestine without being fully processed.

Carbohydrate processing involves enzymatic cleavage of specific linkages within polysaccharides and disaccharides. These enzymes act on substrates that are generally more accessible than proteins and fats, but their efficiency still depends on proper timing and interaction with the intestinal surface. When carbohydrates are presented in forms that allow consistent enzyme contact, breakdown into simple sugars occurs rapidly, and absorption follows. When structural barriers persist or when timing is misaligned, enzymatic action becomes uneven, producing a mixture of fully reduced and partially processed fragments that influence both absorption and microbial activity.

The coordination between these pathways is essential because they share the same environment within the intestine. Enzyme secretion, bile delivery, and motility patterns must accommodate all three macronutrients simultaneously. When upstream signaling is accurate, the system adjusts to the composition of the meal, scaling output and timing to match the demands of each component. When signaling is weak or when substrate preparation is incomplete, this coordination breaks down. One pathway may dominate or require compensation, altering the conditions under which the others operate.

Processing efficiency therefore depends on the alignment of structure, timing, and signaling across all macronutrients. Proteins require unfolding and cleavage, fats require dispersion and emulsification, and carbohydrates require accessible linkages and consistent enzyme interaction. Each pathway builds on the work of the previous stage, and disruptions in one area can influence the others through shared mechanisms of motility, secretion, and substrate availability. When the sequence is aligned, all three pathways operate in concert, producing substrates that can be absorbed with minimal variability. When it is not, each pathway reflects the constraints imposed by upstream failure, and the overall efficiency of digestion declines.

Chapter 10

Bile Flow and Fat Emulsification

Bile flow determines whether dietary fat can be transformed into a form that enzymes can access and the intestine can absorb. Lipids enter the digestive system as large, hydrophobic aggregates that resist interaction with the aqueous environment of the gut. Without structural modification, these aggregates limit enzyme contact and prevent efficient breakdown. Bile changes this condition by dispersing fats into smaller, organized structures that increase surface area and allow lipolytic enzymes to engage. The effectiveness of this process depends on both the availability of bile and the timing of its release relative to the arrival of fat in the small intestine.

Bile is produced continuously but stored and concentrated until it is needed. Its release is triggered by signals that originate as fats move from the stomach into the upper small intestine. These signals coordinate gallbladder contraction with pancreatic enzyme secretion, ensuring that bile and lipases are present at the same time. When this coordination is intact, fats are rapidly dispersed into smaller units, and enzymes can cleave them into components that can be transported across the intestinal lining. The sequence relies on this alignment. Bile must arrive when fats require dispersion, not before and not after.

The structural role of bile is central to fat processing. By organizing lipids into smaller particles, bile increases the interface between fat and the surrounding fluid, creating conditions where enzymes can access and cleave triglycerides effectively. Without this dispersion, lipases encounter large, compact fat masses with limited surface exposure. Enzymatic activity becomes restricted to outer layers, leaving internal portions unprocessed. The difference between dispersed and aggregated fat determines how much of the dietary lipid load can be reduced and absorbed.

Upstream conditions influence how well bile can perform this role. When gastric processing exposes fats and delivers them into the intestine in a controlled manner, bile can interact with substrates that are already positioned for dispersion. When fats arrive in larger aggregates due to incomplete preparation or when gastric emptying is irregular, bile delivery may not align with the substrate. Portions of fat may pass through without adequate emulsification, reducing the efficiency of breakdown and absorption.

Timing remains the critical variable. Signals that regulate bile release depend on the detection of fat within the intestine, but these signals are influenced by earlier stages of digestion. Weak early-phase signaling or disrupted gastric coordination can delay or reduce the strength of these signals, leading to bile release that is insufficient or mistimed. When bile arrives too early, it may not coincide with the presence of fat. When it arrives too late, fats may have already progressed beyond the optimal region for emulsification. In both cases, the interaction between bile and substrate is reduced.

The consequences of impaired bile flow extend beyond fat absorption. Lipids that are not properly processed continue through the intestine, altering the luminal environment and influencing how other nutrients are handled. These unprocessed fats can affect motility and interact with microbial populations, contributing to variability in the digestive sequence. The system attempts to compensate through adjustments in motility and secretion, but these responses do not restore the initial alignment required for efficient fat processing.

Bile flow and fat emulsification therefore represent a coordinated process that depends on structural preparation, signaling, and timing. Bile does not act in isolation. Its effectiveness is determined by how well the system delivers fats into the intestine and how precisely its release is aligned with that delivery. When these elements are synchronized, fat digestion proceeds with consistency. When they are not, the efficiency of lipid processing declines, and the effects propagate through the remainder of the digestive system.

Bile as a Structural Fluid, Not Just Digestive

Bile functions by changing the physical organization of lipids rather than simply assisting in their breakdown. It acts as a structural agent that reorganizes fat within the intestinal environment, converting large, hydrophobic aggregates into dispersed particles that can interact with enzymes and the surrounding fluid. This transformation determines whether lipids can be processed and absorbed. Without it, fats remain in forms that resist enzymatic access and limit transport across the intestinal lining.

The amphipathic nature of bile components allows them to interface between fat and water, creating stable structures that increase surface exposure. As bile interacts with dietary lipids, it breaks larger masses into smaller units and stabilizes them within the aqueous environment of the intestine. This increases the contact area available to lipolytic enzymes, allowing cleavage to occur across a broader surface rather than being confined to the outer layers of a compact fat mass. The structural arrangement created by bile therefore defines the efficiency of enzymatic action.

This role extends beyond initial dispersion. Bile maintains the organization of lipid-derived products after enzymatic cleavage, forming transportable structures that carry these components to the intestinal lining. These structures move through the luminal environment in a way that allows consistent interaction with the absorptive surface. Without this organization, the products of fat digestion would remain poorly distributed, reducing the likelihood of efficient uptake.

The effectiveness of bile as a structural fluid depends on timing and substrate condition. Lipids must be presented in a state that allows bile to interact with them fully, and bile must be available when this interaction is required. When upstream processing has exposed fats and gastric emptying delivers them in controlled amounts, bile can reorganize them efficiently. When fats arrive in large aggregates or when bile release is misaligned, this structural transformation is incomplete. Portions of the lipid load remain resistant to dispersion, and the efficiency of both enzymatic breakdown and absorption declines.

Bile also influences the broader environment of the intestine. By organizing lipids into smaller particles, it affects how contents move, how enzymes distribute, and how other nutrients interact within the same space. This structural influence extends to the consistency of the luminal contents and the pattern of contact between substrates and the intestinal surface. The physical state of the contents is therefore shaped in part by bile activity, linking lipid processing to overall digestive dynamics.

Viewing bile as a structural fluid clarifies its role within the digestive sequence. It does not merely support digestion in a general sense. It determines the physical form of lipids and their derivatives, and that form dictates whether enzymes can act and whether absorption can occur. When this structural function is aligned with upstream preparation and downstream demand, lipid processing proceeds efficiently. When it is not, fats remain in forms that limit interaction, and the effects extend through the remainder of the digestive system.

Emulsification and Micelle Formation

Fat digestion depends on converting large lipid aggregates into dispersed, transportable structures that can move through an aqueous environment and interact with the intestinal surface. Emulsification is the first step in this transformation. Bile interacts with dietary fat and breaks it into smaller droplets, increasing the total surface area exposed to digestive enzymes. This is not a passive mixing process. It is a structural reorganization that changes how lipids behave within the intestinal lumen, allowing them to remain suspended rather than separating into larger, inaccessible masses.

As emulsification progresses, lipolytic enzymes act on the surface of these droplets, cleaving triglycerides into smaller components. These products do not remain randomly distributed. They are incorporated into organized assemblies known as micelles, which are formed through the interaction of bile components with lipid breakdown products. Micelles act as carriers that keep hydrophobic molecules dispersed within the aqueous environment of the intestine. Without this organization, these molecules would tend to re-aggregate, reducing their availability for absorption.

The formation of micelles determines whether lipid-derived components can reach the intestinal lining in a form that can be taken up. These structures move through the luminal space and deliver their contents to the surface of the epithelium, where absorption occurs. The efficiency of this delivery depends on the stability and concentration of micelles. When emulsification is complete and bile availability is sufficient, micelle formation proceeds consistently, and lipid transport to the absorptive surface is maintained.

Upstream conditions influence how effectively this sequence operates. Lipids must be presented in a state that allows bile to interact with them, and the timing of bile release must align with the arrival of fat in the intestine. When gastric processing exposes fats and delivers them in controlled amounts, emulsification occurs efficiently, and micelle formation follows. When fats arrive in larger aggregates or when bile release is delayed or insufficient, emulsification is incomplete. This limits the formation of micelles and reduces the delivery of lipid components to the intestinal lining.

The interaction between emulsification and micelle formation also affects the overall environment within the intestine. Properly dispersed lipids allow enzymes to act uniformly and maintain a consistent pattern of breakdown. When dispersion is incomplete, regions of the lumen contain lipids in different states, creating variability in enzyme activity and transport. This variability influences how effectively nutrients are absorbed and how stable the digestive process remains.

Emulsification and micelle formation therefore represent a continuous structural process that converts dietary fat into absorbable units. The transition from large aggregates to dispersed droplets and then to organized transport structures defines whether lipids can be processed and absorbed efficiently. When this sequence is aligned with upstream preparation and downstream demand, fat digestion proceeds with consistency. When it is disrupted, the physical state of lipids limits interaction at every stage, and the efficiency of the system declines.

Fat Digestion as System Stabilizer

Fat digestion influences the stability of the entire digestive sequence because it directly shapes the timing, signaling, and physical environment within the intestine. Lipids are not processed in isolation. Their presence alters how quickly material moves, how enzymes are released, and how the system coordinates the transition between stages. When fat digestion is aligned, these effects create a controlled, predictable flow through the digestive tract. When it is disrupted, variability increases across multiple processes at once.

The presence of fat slows gastric emptying through coordinated signaling, extending the time available for upstream processing and ensuring that the small intestine receives material in manageable portions. This controlled release allows enzyme activity and bile delivery to remain synchronized with substrate arrival. The intestine operates within a stable range of input, where breakdown and absorption can proceed without being overwhelmed. Fat therefore acts as a pacing mechanism, regulating the speed of the sequence so that each stage has sufficient time to perform its function.

Bile-mediated dispersion of lipids contributes to this stability by organizing the physical state of the luminal contents. When fats are emulsified and incorporated into micelles, they are distributed evenly within the intestinal environment. This uniformity supports consistent enzyme activity and reduces variability in how substrates interact with the intestinal surface. The system processes a more homogeneous mixture, allowing breakdown and absorption to proceed with fewer fluctuations.

Fat digestion also influences hormonal and neural signaling that coordinate digestive activity. The detection of lipids in the intestine generates signals that adjust enzyme secretion, bile flow, and motility patterns. When these signals are aligned with the actual state of the substrate, they reinforce coordination across the system. Enzymes are delivered when needed, bile is released in proportion to fat content, and motility is adjusted to maintain appropriate contact time. These responses create a feedback loop that stabilizes the sequence.

When fat digestion is impaired, this stabilizing effect is lost. Inadequate emulsification or mistimed bile release leaves lipids in forms that resist enzymatic action. These unprocessed fats alter the physical environment, affecting how other nutrients are handled and how contents move through the intestine. The signals that regulate motility and secretion become less reliable because they are based on substrates that do not match expected conditions. The system shifts from coordinated pacing to reactive adjustment, increasing variability in transit and processing.

The influence of fat digestion extends beyond lipid handling alone. Because it regulates timing, distribution, and signaling, it affects how proteins and carbohydrates are processed within the same environment. A stable lipid processing sequence supports consistent conditions for all macronutrients, while disruption in this pathway introduces variability that propagates across the entire system.

Fat digestion therefore acts as a stabilizing force within digestion by controlling the rate and organization of the sequence. When emulsification, enzyme activity, and signaling are aligned, lipids contribute to a steady and coordinated flow that supports efficient breakdown and absorption. When this alignment is lost, the system becomes less predictable, and the effects extend to every component of digestion.

Chapter 11

Absorption and Transport

Absorption is the stage where the products of digestion move from the intestinal lumen into the body's internal environment, but this transfer depends entirely on the form in which those products arrive. The intestinal lining is structured to take up specific molecular forms through defined transport mechanisms. Amino acids, small peptides, simple sugars, and lipid transport structures are handled through pathways that require prior reduction and organization. When digestion has proceeded with proper sequencing, these forms are present in consistent quantities, and absorption operates as a continuous, efficient process. When upstream breakdown is incomplete, the available substrates do not match these transport systems, and the movement of nutrients across the intestinal barrier becomes limited and uneven.

The surface of the small intestine is organized to maximize contact between luminal contents and absorptive cells. This structure allows for high-capacity uptake when substrates are in their intended forms. Transport proteins within these cells move nutrients across the epithelial layer, and this movement depends on both concentration gradients and the availability of compatible substrates. When peptides and amino acids are present in sufficient amounts, protein-derived nutrients are taken up efficiently. When carbohydrates are fully reduced to simple sugars, their transport proceeds rapidly. When lipid-derived components are organized into micelles and related structures, they can approach the epithelial surface and be absorbed.

The transition from the lumen into the cell requires that substrates be both chemically and physically prepared. Larger fragments or poorly organized molecules do not engage transport systems effectively. They remain within the lumen or move forward without being absorbed. This creates a situation where the presence of nutrients does not translate into uptake because the structural requirements for transport have not been met. The efficiency of absorption is therefore determined upstream, at the level of digestion, rather than at the level of the transport mechanism itself.

Once nutrients cross the epithelial layer, they enter distribution pathways that deliver them to different regions of the body. Water-soluble components move into the circulation, while lipid-derived components follow a pathway that reflects their hydrophobic nature. These transport routes depend on the initial form in which nutrients are absorbed. When absorption is consistent, distribution proceeds with predictable patterns, supplying tissues with the substrates required for energy production, structural maintenance, and signaling. When absorption is uneven, distribution becomes variable, and the availability of nutrients at the tissue level fluctuates.

The coordination between absorption and transport also depends on timing. Nutrients must be absorbed in a pattern that aligns with their arrival in the intestine. When gastric emptying and intestinal motility are consistent, substrates are presented to the absorptive surface in a steady flow, allowing transport systems to operate continuously. When upstream processes are irregular, substrates arrive in pulses or in forms that vary in readiness for absorption. This disrupts the continuity of uptake and introduces variability into the transport phase.

Absorption is therefore not a passive endpoint but an active process that reflects the entire sequence that precedes it. The structure of the intestinal lining and its transport mechanisms are designed to operate on substrates that have been properly prepared. When this preparation is achieved, absorption and transport proceed with stability and efficiency. When it is not, the system encounters substrates that it cannot fully utilize, and the movement of nutrients into the body becomes constrained by the conditions established earlier in digestion.

Membrane Transport Systems

Membrane transport systems determine which digestion products actually enter the body and at what rate, and they operate with strict structural requirements. The intestinal epithelium is not a passive surface that absorbs anything present in the lumen. It is a selectively gated interface built from lipid membranes embedded with transport proteins, each designed to move specific molecular forms across the barrier. These systems recognize size, charge, and configuration. When substrates match these parameters, transport proceeds efficiently. When they do not, the substrate remains in the lumen regardless of how much is present.

Protein-derived nutrients are absorbed through transporters that move amino acids and small peptides across the epithelial membrane. These systems require proteins to be reduced to a defined range of sizes. Dipeptides, tripeptides, and individual amino acids are compatible with transport mechanisms that move them into the cell. Larger fragments do not engage these systems effectively. They remain outside the membrane, continuing along the intestine or interacting with the epithelial surface in ways that can trigger secondary responses. The limitation is not the number of transporters. It is the structural form of the substrate presented to them.

Carbohydrate transport follows a similar pattern. Specific transporters move simple sugars across the membrane, relying on concentration gradients and cellular energy to drive uptake. These transporters do not process complex carbohydrates directly. The substrate must be reduced to monosaccharides before it can be absorbed. When breakdown is complete, transport is rapid and consistent. When reduction is incomplete, fragments that cannot engage these transporters persist within the lumen, contributing to variability in both absorption and downstream microbial activity.

Lipid transport introduces an additional layer of structural dependency. Fat-derived components must be organized into micelles to approach the epithelial surface, and once inside the cell, they are reassembled into transportable forms that can move through the body. This process depends on the prior action of bile and lipolytic enzymes. Without proper emulsification and breakdown, lipid components do not reach the membrane in a form that can be taken up. The membrane itself, composed of lipid bilayers, interacts with these substrates in a way that reflects their structural compatibility. Properly organized lipid products integrate into this system, while poorly prepared aggregates do not.

The membrane environment itself influences transport efficiency. The composition of the epithelial membrane, including its lipid structure, affects fluidity and the function of embedded transport proteins.

This structure determines how easily substrates can interact with and pass through the membrane. When the membrane is operating within its intended parameters, transport systems function with predictable capacity. When the internal environment is altered, the behavior of these systems can shift, affecting the rate and consistency of nutrient uptake.

Timing and concentration also shape how these transport systems operate. A steady delivery of properly prepared substrates allows transporters to function continuously, maintaining consistent uptake. When substrates arrive in irregular pulses or in mixed states of readiness, transport becomes uneven. Periods of high availability may be followed by periods where compatible substrates are limited, reducing overall efficiency. The system responds to these fluctuations, but the variability originates from upstream conditions rather than from the transport mechanisms themselves.

Membrane transport systems therefore act as the final filter in the digestive sequence, enforcing structural requirements that reflect the design of the system. They do not compensate for incomplete digestion. They accept substrates that meet their criteria and exclude those that do not. The effectiveness of absorption is determined by how well upstream processes produce the forms that these systems are built to handle.

Chylomicrons and Lipid Delivery

Lipid absorption does not end at the intestinal membrane. Once fatty acids and related components enter the epithelial cell, they are reorganized into larger transport structures that can move through the body without disrupting the aqueous environment of the circulation. Chylomicrons are the primary carriers that perform this function. They package lipid components into a form that can be distributed to tissues while maintaining compatibility with the fluid systems that transport them.

Inside the intestinal cell, absorbed lipid components are reassembled into triglycerides and combined with structural molecules that stabilize the particle. This assembly creates a spherical structure with a lipid core and a surface that allows it to remain suspended in fluid. The formation of chylomicrons depends on the prior steps of digestion and absorption. Lipids must be reduced to forms that can cross the membrane, and those components must then be available in sufficient quantity to be repackaged. When upstream processes are aligned, this assembly occurs efficiently, producing particles that can be released into the transport system.

Chylomicrons do not enter the bloodstream directly. They move into the lymphatic system, which provides a pathway suited to transporting large lipid-rich particles. This route allows lipids to be distributed without overwhelming the immediate circulatory environment. From the lymphatic system, chylomicrons eventually enter the bloodstream, where they deliver their lipid content to tissues that require it for energy, membrane structure, and signaling processes.

The structure of chylomicrons determines how lipids are delivered. Their size and composition allow them to interact with enzymes and tissues in a controlled manner, releasing fatty acids where they are needed. This process depends on the integrity of the particle. When chylomicrons are properly formed, lipid delivery is gradual and coordinated. When formation is impaired due to incomplete digestion or absorption, fewer particles are produced, and lipid distribution becomes limited.

The efficiency of this system is tied to earlier stages of fat processing. Emulsification, enzymatic breakdown, and micelle formation all determine how much lipid reaches the epithelial cell in a form that can be absorbed. If these steps are incomplete, the pool of available components for chylomicron assembly is reduced. This limits the amount of lipid that can be packaged and transported, affecting the supply of these molecules to the rest of the body.

Chylomicron formation also influences the timing of lipid delivery. Because these particles move through the lymphatic system before entering the bloodstream, lipid distribution occurs over a longer time frame compared to water-soluble nutrients. This extended delivery contributes to the regulation of energy availability and supports sustained metabolic activity. When formation is consistent, lipid supply is steady. When it is disrupted, delivery becomes irregular.

Chylomicrons therefore serve as the link between intestinal absorption and systemic lipid distribution. They convert absorbed lipid components into a transportable form that can move through the body without disrupting fluid balance. Their formation and function depend on the alignment of upstream digestive processes, and their effectiveness reflects how well those processes have prepared and delivered lipid substrates to the point of absorption.

Nutrient Allocation vs Simple Absorption

Absorption describes the movement of nutrients across the intestinal membrane, but allocation determines where those nutrients go, how quickly they are used, and whether they are stored or oxidized. These are not the same process. The intestine can transfer substrates into the body while allocation pathways decide their fate within circulation and tissues. A system can absorb nutrients effectively and still distribute them in ways that do not match current demands. The outcome depends on signaling, transport structure, and the condition of the receiving tissues.

Water-soluble nutrients enter the bloodstream and are distributed according to concentration gradients and tissue uptake signals. Glucose and amino acids move rapidly through circulation, and their allocation depends on hormonal signals that control uptake and storage. When tissues are primed to receive these substrates, transport into cells proceeds efficiently. When signaling is altered, these nutrients remain in circulation longer or are redirected toward storage pathways. The presence of nutrients in the blood does not guarantee their use. Allocation determines whether they are oxidized for energy, incorporated into structural components, or stored.

Lipid-derived nutrients follow a different route that reflects their physical properties. Chylomicrons carry these lipids through the lymphatic system and into circulation, where they are gradually delivered to tissues. This staged release creates a delayed and sustained allocation pattern compared to water-soluble nutrients. The distribution of lipids depends on tissue demand and enzymatic activity that governs the release of fatty acids from transport particles. When this system is aligned, lipids are delivered in a controlled manner that supports membrane structure, energy production, and signaling functions.

Allocation is influenced by the condition of the digestive sequence that precedes it. When digestion and absorption produce consistent substrate forms, transport and distribution follow predictable patterns. When upstream processes are irregular, the timing and composition of absorbed nutrients vary. This variability carries forward into allocation, where tissues receive substrates in inconsistent amounts or at inappropriate times. The system adapts to these fluctuations, but the stability of distribution is reduced.

The distinction between absorption and allocation becomes clear when considering capacity. Absorption capacity is defined by transport systems at the intestinal level, while allocation capacity is defined by how tissues receive and process incoming substrates. If tissues are not prepared to use a given nutrient, it may be stored or remain in circulation. This can occur even when absorption is functioning normally. The system must align both processes to maintain efficient use of nutrients.

Hormonal and neural signals coordinate allocation by linking nutrient availability to tissue demand. These signals adjust uptake rates, storage pathways, and energy utilization. When they are aligned with the actual condition of the body, allocation supports stable metabolic function. When they are not, nutrients are distributed in ways that do not match current needs, leading to inefficiencies in energy use and structural maintenance.

Nutrient allocation therefore extends beyond the act of absorption. It determines how the products of digestion are integrated into the body's systems. Absorption moves substrates into circulation, but allocation governs their distribution, timing, and use. The effectiveness of this process reflects both the quality of upstream digestion and the state of the tissues that receive these nutrients.

PART VI

LIPID DIGESTION AS SYSTEM CONTROL

Chapter 12

Fat as a Digestive Regulator

Fat enters the digestive system as more than a caloric substrate. It acts as a regulatory input that shapes the timing, coordination, and physical behavior of the entire sequence. The presence of lipid in the stomach and small intestine alters how quickly material moves, how strongly digestive secretions are released, and how downstream stages prepare for incoming substrates. These effects are not secondary. They define the operating conditions under which digestion proceeds, determining whether the sequence remains controlled or becomes variable.

When fat reaches the upper small intestine, it generates signaling that slows gastric emptying. This delay is not incidental. It extends the time available for gastric processing and ensures that the intestine receives material in portions that match its capacity. The stomach releases its contents more gradually, allowing bile flow and enzyme secretion to align with substrate arrival. This pacing function stabilizes the sequence. Instead of rapid delivery followed by overload, the system maintains a controlled flow that supports consistent breakdown and absorption.

Fat also influences the strength and coordination of digestive secretions. The detection of lipid within the intestine triggers the release of bile and pancreatic enzymes in proportion to the amount of fat present. This creates a feedback system where substrate presence drives the availability of the tools required to process it. When fat digestion is aligned, this signaling produces a balanced environment in which dispersion, enzymatic breakdown, and absorption occur together. When lipid signaling is weak or mistimed, these processes become uncoupled, and efficiency declines.

The structural effects of fat further contribute to its regulatory role. Lipids alter the physical state of luminal contents, affecting viscosity, mixing patterns, and contact with the intestinal surface. When fats are properly emulsified, they form a dispersed system that supports uniform enzyme activity and consistent interaction with the epithelium. This reduces variability in how substrates are processed across different regions of the intestine. When emulsification is incomplete, fats remain in larger aggregates, disrupting this uniformity and creating localized differences in digestion.

Fat also interacts with motility patterns along the digestive tract. Its presence modifies the rhythm and intensity of intestinal contractions, influencing how contents move and how long they remain in contact with absorptive surfaces. When lipid signaling is aligned with substrate condition, motility supports efficient progression without excessive speed or delay. When signaling is disrupted, motility becomes less predictable, contributing to irregular transit times and inconsistent processing.

The regulatory role of fat extends into the coordination of nutrient handling beyond lipids themselves. By controlling pacing, secretion, and motility, fat indirectly influences how proteins and carbohydrates are processed within the same environment. A stable lipid-driven sequence supports consistent conditions for all macronutrients, while disruption in fat processing introduces variability that affects the entire system.

Fat therefore functions as a central regulator of digestion, shaping the sequence through its effects on timing, signaling, and structure. Its influence is expressed through coordinated changes in gastric emptying, enzyme release, bile flow, and motility. When these elements are aligned, fat supports a stable and efficient digestive process. When they are not, the regulatory control it provides is diminished, and variability propagates through the system.

Fat Digestion as the Organizer of Gut Stability

Fat digestion organizes the digestive tract by setting the pace, shaping the physical state of luminal contents, and aligning secretion with substrate demand. When lipids enter the upper intestine in a form that can be dispersed, they trigger coordinated responses that slow gastric output, increase bile flow, and scale pancreatic enzyme delivery to the amount of fat present. This creates a controlled inflow rather than a surge. The intestine receives material at a rate it can process, and the system operates within a stable range where breakdown and absorption remain continuous instead of intermittent.

The structural transformation of lipids drives this stability. Emulsification converts large fat aggregates into smaller droplets, and micelle formation maintains those products in a dispersed state. This uniform distribution changes how enzymes interact with substrates and how contents contact the epithelial surface. Enzymatic activity becomes more evenly distributed across the lumen, reducing regions of under-processing and overloading. The intestine works on a consistent mixture rather than on pockets of dense substrate separated by relatively empty fluid. That uniformity stabilizes both the rate of breakdown and the pattern of absorption.

Signal strength and timing follow the same pattern. Lipid presence generates feedback that links substrate arrival to secretion. When fat is properly processed upstream and delivered in controlled amounts, bile and enzymes are released in proportion to need, and motility adjusts to maintain contact time. The sequence stays synchronized because each stage is responding to inputs that match its operating conditions. When fat digestion is impaired, this coupling weakens. Signals are generated from substrates that are poorly dispersed or inconsistently delivered, so secretion and motility no longer align with what is actually present in the lumen.

Motility reflects this organization. With intact lipid signaling, intestinal contractions maintain a steady progression that supports mixing without accelerating transit beyond processing capacity. The contents remain in contact with enzymes and the epithelial surface long enough for reduction and uptake to occur. When lipid processing is incomplete, motility patterns become less predictable. Portions of the lumen move too quickly while others retain material longer, and the distribution of substrates becomes uneven. This variability feeds back into secretion and absorption, amplifying inconsistency across the system.

The stabilizing effect of fat digestion extends to other nutrients because it defines the environment in which they are processed. Proteins and carbohydrates are exposed to enzymes within the same luminal space shaped by lipid dispersion and pacing. When fat digestion is aligned, these substrates are presented under steady conditions, and their breakdown follows a predictable course. When lipid processing is disrupted, the physical and temporal environment shifts, and protein and carbohydrate handling becomes more variable.

Fat digestion therefore acts as the organizing force of gut stability by controlling flow, structure, and signaling at the same time. It determines whether the digestive sequence operates as a coordinated system or as a set of reactive adjustments. When emulsification, enzyme activity, and bile delivery are aligned with substrate arrival, the intestine processes a stable input and maintains consistent output. When that alignment is lost, variability increases at every stage, and the system moves away from coordinated function.

Lipid Digestion and Food Tolerance

Food tolerance reflects the system's ability to take in a mixed meal, reduce it into defined molecular forms, and move those forms across the intestinal barrier without triggering disruption in motility, fermentation, or immune activity. Lipid digestion sits at the center of this capacity because it sets the conditions under which other macronutrients are processed. When fats are dispersed, matched with bile and enzymes, and delivered at a controlled rate, the intestine operates within a stable range where proteins and carbohydrates can be reduced and absorbed without accumulating in the lumen. When lipid processing is incomplete or mistimed, that stability breaks, and tolerance narrows.

The first effect appears in pacing. Lipids slow gastric emptying and meter the flow of chyme into the small intestine. This controlled delivery prevents sudden increases in substrate load that exceed enzymatic capacity. When fat digestion is aligned, proteins and carbohydrates arrive alongside a steady supply of bile and pancreatic enzymes, and reduction proceeds without backlog. When lipid signaling is weak or delayed, gastric output becomes less regulated, and larger pulses of partially processed material reach the intestine. Enzymes and bile are then forced to react to a load that has already arrived, creating periods where substrate exceeds processing capacity.

The physical state of luminal contents follows the same pattern. Effective emulsification distributes lipids into small droplets and maintains breakdown products in micellar structures. This creates a uniform mixture where enzymes can access substrates consistently and where contact with the epithelial surface is even across the lumen. Proteins and carbohydrates are exposed to a stable environment with predictable mixing. When fats remain in larger aggregates, regions of the intestine contain concentrated substrate while adjacent areas are relatively dilute. Enzymatic activity becomes uneven, and portions of protein and carbohydrate remain only partially reduced as they move forward.

These upstream differences determine what reaches the distal intestine. When digestion is aligned, most substrates have been reduced to forms compatible with membrane transport, and the remaining material is limited. When lipid processing is impaired, a greater fraction of protein and carbohydrate arrives in larger fragments. These fragments interact with the resident microbiota, increasing fermentation and gas production, and they alter the chemical environment within the lumen. Motility adjusts in response to these changes, but the adjustment is reactive and often increases variability in transit.

Immune exposure is shaped by the same sequence. The epithelial barrier is designed to encounter nutrients in specific molecular forms. When proteins are reduced to small peptides and amino acids, interaction with the immune system remains controlled. When larger fragments persist due to incomplete digestion, contact with the epithelial surface increases, and signaling within the mucosal immune system rises. The result is not a single reaction to a specific food but a pattern of sensitivity that follows the state of digestion. The same food may be tolerated under one set of conditions and provoke symptoms under another.

Lipid digestion therefore sets the boundaries of food tolerance by controlling flow, structure, and downstream substrate availability. It determines whether the intestine processes a steady, uniform input or receives irregular loads that exceed local capacity. When emulsification, enzyme activity, and bile delivery are aligned with substrate arrival, proteins and carbohydrates are reduced efficiently, microbial fermentation remains limited, and immune exposure is constrained. When that alignment is lost, partially processed material accumulates, fermentation increases, and tolerance narrows as the system shifts from coordinated processing to reactive adjustment.

Gut Environment Stabilization Through Fats

The internal environment of the intestine is not fixed. It is continuously shaped by the composition, structure, and timing of the material moving through it. Fats play a central role in stabilizing this environment because they influence how contents are distributed, how quickly they move, and how secretions are coordinated with substrate presence. When lipid digestion is aligned, the intestine operates under steady conditions where enzyme activity, motility, and absorption occur in a predictable pattern. When it is not, the internal environment becomes uneven, and variability increases across the system.

The first stabilizing effect appears in the physical organization of luminal contents. Emulsified fats create a dispersed mixture that supports uniform distribution of substrates. This prevents the formation of dense pockets of undigested material that would otherwise concentrate enzymatic activity in some regions while leaving others underprocessed. A uniform mixture allows enzymes to act across the entire volume of contents, maintaining consistency in breakdown. This structural stability reduces fluctuations in how nutrients are processed as they move through the intestine.

Fats also regulate the rate at which material enters and moves through the digestive tract. By slowing gastric emptying, lipids control the initial delivery of substrates into the small intestine. This pacing ensures that the intestine receives a continuous flow rather than intermittent surges. Motility patterns adjust to this steady input, maintaining contact time between substrates and the epithelial surface. When this pacing is intact, the system avoids both overload and rapid transit, supporting consistent processing and absorption.

The coordination of digestive secretions depends on the presence of fats as well. Lipids trigger the release of bile and pancreatic enzymes in proportion to their concentration, aligning the availability of these secretions with the amount of substrate present. This creates a feedback system where the environment adapts to match incoming material. When lipid signaling is consistent, bile flow and enzyme activity remain synchronized with digestion, maintaining stable conditions within the lumen. When signaling is disrupted, secretion patterns become less aligned, contributing to variability in the internal environment.

The chemical conditions within the intestine are also influenced by fat digestion. Proper emulsification and breakdown limit the amount of unprocessed substrate that reaches later sections of the intestine. This reduces the variability in microbial activity and the production of fermentation byproducts, which can alter the local environment. When lipid digestion is impaired, more undigested material progresses downstream, changing the composition of the luminal contents and increasing fluctuations in chemical conditions.

Fats therefore stabilize the gut environment by controlling structure, flow, and signaling at the same time. They determine how evenly substrates are distributed, how steadily they are delivered, and how precisely the system responds to their presence. When lipid digestion is aligned with the rest of the digestive sequence, the intestine operates within a narrow and predictable range of conditions. When it is not, the environment becomes less stable, and the effects extend to every stage of digestion and absorption.

Chapter 13

Fat-Soluble Nutrients as Outputs

Fat-soluble nutrients emerge from digestion as the result of a sequence that has successfully reduced, organized, and transported lipid-associated compounds into forms that can be absorbed and delivered to tissues. These nutrients do not enter the system independently. They are carried within the same structures that handle dietary fat, and their availability depends on how well lipid digestion has been executed. When emulsification, enzymatic breakdown, and micelle formation are aligned, these compounds move through the intestine in a form that can reach the epithelial surface and cross into the body. When lipid processing is incomplete, their presence in the diet does not translate into absorption.

The defining feature of fat-soluble nutrients is their dependence on lipid transport structures. They associate with dietary fats during digestion and are incorporated into the same micellar systems that carry lipid breakdown products. This association allows them to remain dispersed within the aqueous environment of the intestine and approach the absorptive surface. Without this structural integration, these compounds remain in the lumen, unable to engage the transport systems that move them into the body. Their absorption is therefore determined by the same conditions that govern fat processing.

Once inside the epithelial cell, these nutrients are incorporated into the lipid transport pathway that leads to chylomicron formation. This step packages them into particles that can move through the lymphatic system and eventually enter circulation. The distribution of fat-soluble nutrients follows the same route as lipid-derived energy substrates, linking their delivery to the broader system of lipid transport. When this pathway is functioning consistently, these nutrients are distributed to tissues in a controlled manner that supports structural and signaling functions.

The availability of fat-soluble nutrients at the tissue level reflects both their intake and the efficiency of the digestive sequence. When lipid digestion is aligned, these compounds are absorbed in proportion to their presence in the diet and delivered through established transport pathways. When lipid processing is impaired, their absorption is reduced regardless of intake. Increasing dietary supply does not compensate for a failure in the structural and transport systems required for their uptake.

Timing also influences how these nutrients are delivered. Because they are transported within chylomicrons, their entry into circulation occurs over a longer period compared to water-soluble nutrients. This extended delivery supports sustained availability, allowing tissues to access these compounds over time. When chylomicron formation is consistent, this distribution pattern remains stable. When it is disrupted, delivery becomes irregular, and tissue access to these nutrients fluctuates.

Fat-soluble nutrients therefore represent outputs of a functioning lipid digestion system rather than isolated inputs. Their presence within the body depends on the alignment of upstream processes that prepare and transport them. When the sequence is intact, these nutrients are absorbed and distributed in a manner that supports cellular structure and signaling. When it is not, their movement into the body is constrained by the same factors that limit lipid digestion, and their functional availability declines.

Vitamins A, D, E, K as Digestion-Dependent

Vitamins A, D, E, and K enter the digestive tract bound to dietary fat and remain dependent on lipid processing at every stage of their movement into the body. They do not dissolve freely in the aqueous environment of the intestine, and they cannot approach the epithelial surface or cross the membrane without being incorporated into lipid transport structures. Their absorption is therefore determined by the same sequence that governs fat digestion, including emulsification, enzymatic breakdown, micelle formation, and chylomicron assembly. When this sequence is intact, these vitamins move with dietary lipids and become available to tissues. When it is not, they remain within the lumen and are lost regardless of intake.

The first requirement for their absorption is dispersion. As bile interacts with dietary fats, it creates a system in which lipid-associated compounds can remain suspended and accessible. Vitamins A, D, E, and K are incorporated into these dispersed structures, allowing them to move through the intestinal environment without separating from the lipid phase. This step determines whether they can reach the epithelial surface. Without adequate emulsification, these vitamins remain within larger fat aggregates that limit their exposure to the absorptive interface.

Micelle formation extends this process by organizing lipid breakdown products and associated compounds into transportable units. These structures carry fat-soluble vitamins to the surface of the intestinal cells, positioning them for uptake. The stability and concentration of micelles determine how effectively these vitamins are delivered. When micelle formation is consistent, delivery is continuous and absorption proceeds in proportion to dietary supply. When it is reduced, the movement of these vitamins toward the epithelial surface is limited, and their uptake declines.

Once inside the epithelial cell, these vitamins are incorporated into chylomicrons along with reassembled lipids. This packaging step determines their distribution through the body. Chylomicrons move through the lymphatic system and into circulation, delivering lipid-associated compounds to tissues over time. The efficiency of this process depends on the availability of lipid components within the cell and the integrity of the assembly pathway. When upstream digestion provides a consistent supply of absorbable lipid substrates, chylomicron formation supports stable delivery of these vitamins. When that supply is reduced, their transport is limited.

The dependence of vitamins A, D, E, and K on lipid digestion means that their functional availability reflects digestive capacity rather than intake alone. A diet containing sufficient amounts of these nutrients does not ensure their absorption if the structural and transport processes required for lipid handling are impaired. Increasing intake under these conditions does not resolve the limitation because the constraint lies in the system that processes and moves them, not in the amount present in the lumen.

The timing of lipid digestion also influences their delivery. Because these vitamins travel within chylomicrons, their entry into circulation follows the same delayed pattern as lipid-derived substrates. This creates a sustained distribution over time, allowing tissues to access them gradually. When digestion and transport are consistent, this pattern supports stable availability. When they are not, delivery becomes irregular, and tissue levels fluctuate.

Vitamins A, D, E, and K therefore function as outputs of a coordinated lipid digestion system. Their absorption and transport depend on the structural transformations that occur during fat processing and the pathways that carry lipids through the body. When these processes are aligned, these vitamins are absorbed and distributed in a manner that supports their roles in cellular function. When they are not, their movement into the body is constrained by the same factors that limit lipid digestion, and their availability is reduced despite adequate intake.

Bile-Mediated Absorption

Bile determines whether lipid-derived substrates and fat-soluble compounds reach the intestinal membrane in a form that can be absorbed. It does this by organizing hydrophobic molecules into transportable structures that can exist within the aqueous environment of the lumen. Without this organization, lipids and associated nutrients remain separated from the epithelial surface, limiting interaction with transport systems. Absorption is therefore not driven by the presence of these molecules alone, but by their structural integration into bile-dependent assemblies that can move through the intestinal space and present themselves for uptake.

The process begins with dispersion. Bile interacts with incoming lipids and breaks them into smaller units, increasing the interface between fat and the surrounding fluid. This change in physical structure allows enzymes to act more effectively, generating smaller lipid components that can be incorporated into micellar structures. These micelles act as carriers that keep lipid-derived molecules suspended and mobile within the lumen. They move toward the epithelial surface, maintaining contact between hydrophobic substrates and the absorptive interface.

The delivery of substrates to the membrane depends on the stability and concentration of these bile-driven structures. When bile flow is sufficient and aligned with substrate arrival, micelles form in adequate numbers and persist long enough to deliver their contents to the epithelial surface. This creates a continuous supply of absorbable material, allowing transport systems to operate at a steady rate. When bile availability is reduced or mistimed, micelle formation declines. Lipid-derived molecules remain dispersed unevenly or re-aggregate, limiting their movement toward the membrane and reducing absorption.

Bile-mediated absorption also determines the uptake of fat-soluble nutrients. Vitamins and other lipid-associated compounds are carried within the same micellar structures as fatty acids and monoglycerides. Their delivery to the epithelial surface depends on the same process of dispersion and organization. When bile activity is aligned, these compounds move efficiently toward the membrane and are absorbed alongside lipid breakdown products. When it is not, their delivery is restricted, and their uptake declines regardless of their presence in the intestinal contents.

The interaction between micelles and the epithelial membrane reflects both the structure of the substrate and the condition of the membrane itself. Micelles bring lipid-derived molecules into proximity with the membrane, where they can be transferred into the cell. This transfer depends on the compatibility between the substrate and the lipid environment of the membrane. When substrates are properly organized, this interaction proceeds efficiently. When they are not, transfer is limited, and absorption remains incomplete.

Bile-mediated absorption therefore represents the final step in converting lipid-derived molecules from luminal contents into intracellular substrates. It links the structural reorganization of fats to their movement across the epithelial barrier. The effectiveness of this process depends on the alignment of bile flow, substrate condition, and timing. When these elements are coordinated, absorption proceeds continuously. When they are not, the delivery of substrates to the membrane is reduced, and the movement of lipid-derived nutrients into the body is constrained.

Deficiency as a Delivery Failure, Not Intake Failure

Deficiency emerges when nutrients fail to reach tissues in usable form, not simply when intake is low. The digestive system can contain adequate amounts of a nutrient while the body remains functionally deprived because the processes that move that nutrient from the lumen to the cell are impaired. Absorption, transport, and allocation determine whether a nutrient becomes available to the systems that depend on it. When any part of this sequence is disrupted, intake and tissue availability separate, and deficiency develops despite the presence of sufficient dietary supply.

The first point of failure occurs at the level of digestion. Nutrients must be reduced and organized into forms that can engage transport systems. Fat-soluble compounds require emulsification and micelle formation, while proteins and carbohydrates must be broken into defined molecular units. When this preparation is incomplete, substrates remain in forms that cannot cross the intestinal membrane. They pass through the system without contributing to cellular function. The limitation is not the amount consumed but the inability to convert that intake into absorbable structure.

Transport across the intestinal membrane introduces a second constraint. Membrane transport systems accept only specific molecular configurations, and they operate within defined capacities. When substrates arrive in compatible forms, uptake proceeds efficiently. When they do not, transport is limited regardless of concentration within the lumen. A high intake of a nutrient does not overcome a mismatch between substrate form and transport mechanism. The system enforces structural requirements that determine whether movement into the body occurs.

Once nutrients enter the body, distribution pathways determine whether they reach the tissues that require them. Lipid-derived nutrients depend on chylomicron formation and lymphatic transport, while water-soluble compounds move through circulation under the control of signaling systems that regulate uptake. When these pathways are functioning consistently, nutrients are delivered in a pattern that supports cellular processes. When they are not, distribution becomes uneven. Nutrients may remain in circulation, be redirected to storage, or fail to reach specific tissues in sufficient amounts.

Allocation within tissues represents the final stage of this sequence. Cells must be able to take up and use incoming substrates. This depends on local signaling and metabolic state. When tissues are prepared to receive and utilize nutrients, allocation proceeds effectively. When they are not, nutrients may accumulate without being integrated into functional processes. The presence of a nutrient in circulation does not guarantee its use within the cell.

Deficiency therefore reflects a failure of delivery across multiple stages rather than a simple absence of intake. It arises when digestion does not produce absorbable forms, when transport systems cannot move those forms across the membrane, when distribution pathways fail to deliver them to tissues, or when cellular uptake is impaired. Each of these points can limit availability independently of how much of a nutrient is consumed.

Understanding deficiency in this way shifts the focus from quantity to sequence. Increasing intake does not resolve a delivery failure because the constraint lies in the processes that move and allocate nutrients. Restoring function requires aligning digestion, transport, and distribution so that nutrients can progress through the system and reach the tissues that depend on them.

Chapter 14

Hormones and Lipid Transport

Lipid transport is directed by hormonal signals that determine when fats are stored, when they are released, and how they are distributed between tissues. After lipids are absorbed and packaged into chylomicrons, they enter circulation in a form that requires further regulation before they can be used. Hormones act on both the transport particles and the receiving tissues, controlling the rate at which fatty acids are extracted and the destinations to which they are delivered. This regulation links digestion to systemic energy use and structural maintenance.

Insulin plays a central role in directing lipid flow after a meal. When nutrient availability rises, insulin signals tissues to take up incoming substrates and promotes the storage of fatty acids. It increases the activity of enzymes that allow tissues to extract lipids from circulating particles and incorporate them into storage or structural pools. This process reduces circulating lipid levels and shifts the system toward storage. The strength and duration of this signal determine how much of the incoming lipid load is retained within tissues.

Counter-regulatory signals shift the system in the opposite direction. When energy demand increases or when nutrient availability declines, hormonal signals promote the release of stored lipids and reduce the uptake of new ones. This change alters how transport particles are processed, allowing fatty acids to remain available for use in energy production. The balance between these signals determines whether lipids are directed toward storage or toward immediate utilization.

The interaction between hormones and lipid transport particles controls how quickly lipids are cleared from circulation. Chylomicrons deliver fatty acids to tissues through enzyme-mediated processes that are influenced by hormonal state. When signals favor uptake, these particles are processed rapidly, and their contents are transferred into cells. When signals reduce uptake, the clearance of these particles slows, and lipids remain in circulation longer. This change affects both the timing and distribution of lipid delivery.

Hormonal control also influences how different tissues receive lipids. Some tissues increase uptake under specific conditions, while others reduce it, creating a distribution pattern that reflects current physiological needs. This selective allocation ensures that lipids are delivered to areas where they can be used for energy, membrane structure, or signaling functions. When hormonal signaling is aligned with tissue demand, this distribution remains coordinated. When it is not, lipids may be directed toward storage even when immediate use is required, or remain in circulation without being effectively utilized.

The coordination between digestion and hormonal regulation determines how efficiently lipids move from intake to use. Digestion prepares and delivers lipid substrates into circulation, while hormones direct their fate within the body. When these processes are aligned, lipid transport supports stable energy availability and structural maintenance. When they are not, the movement of lipids becomes less predictable, and their distribution no longer reflects the needs of the system.

Hormones therefore act as the control layer that governs lipid transport beyond the intestine. They translate nutrient availability into directed movement and allocation, shaping how lipids are stored, released, and used. The effectiveness of this system depends on both the integrity of digestive processes and the accuracy of the signals that regulate distribution.

Cholesterol and Hormone Synthesis

Cholesterol functions as a structural precursor for a range of signaling molecules that control growth, metabolism, and stress responses. Its role begins at the level of membrane architecture, where it contributes to stability and fluidity, but extends into the synthesis of steroid hormones that regulate systemic behavior. This dual function links lipid transport and cellular structure to endocrine output. The availability of cholesterol within cells determines whether hormone synthesis can proceed at a rate that matches physiological demand.

Cells acquire cholesterol through both internal production and external delivery. Lipoprotein particles circulating in the bloodstream carry cholesterol to tissues, where it is taken up and incorporated into cellular structures or directed toward synthesis pathways. The balance between uptake and internal synthesis determines the intracellular pool available for hormone production. When delivery is consistent and aligned with demand, cells maintain a stable supply that supports both membrane integrity and signaling functions.

Hormone synthesis begins when cholesterol is transported into specific regions within the cell where enzymatic conversion can occur. This movement represents a controlled step that determines how much substrate enters the synthesis pathway. Once positioned, cholesterol is converted into intermediate molecules that are further processed into active hormones. Each step depends on enzyme availability and cellular conditions, but the entire sequence is limited by the initial supply of cholesterol.

The production of steroid hormones depends on the rate at which cholesterol can be mobilized and converted. When supply is sufficient and transport within the cell is efficient, hormone synthesis can respond to changes in physiological demand. When cholesterol availability is reduced or when its movement into the synthesis pathway is constrained, production declines. This limitation affects the output of hormones that regulate metabolism, stress response, and reproductive function.

Cholesterol transport within the body also influences where hormone synthesis occurs. Different tissues specialize in producing specific hormones, and their ability to do so depends on the delivery of cholesterol through circulating lipoproteins. When lipid transport systems are functioning consistently, these tissues receive a steady supply of substrate. When transport is disrupted, cholesterol delivery becomes uneven, and hormone production can vary between tissues.

The connection between digestion, lipid transport, and hormone synthesis becomes apparent when considering how cholesterol enters the system. Dietary fats influence the formation of lipoproteins that carry cholesterol through the bloodstream, and the efficiency of fat digestion affects how these particles are assembled. When lipid processing is aligned, cholesterol is packaged and delivered in a manner that supports stable distribution. When it is not, the availability of cholesterol for cellular use becomes less predictable.

Cholesterol therefore serves as a central substrate linking lipid transport to endocrine function. Its movement from digestion to circulation and into cells determines whether hormone synthesis can proceed effectively. When delivery, uptake, and intracellular transport are aligned, cholesterol supports both structural and signaling roles. When any part of this sequence is disrupted, hormone production reflects that limitation, and the effects extend across multiple physiological systems.

Lipid-Based Signaling Systems

Lipid-based signaling emerges from the same structural framework that governs membrane composition and lipid transport. Signals are not generated in isolation. They arise from the physical state of membranes, the availability of specific lipid substrates, and the enzymes that convert those substrates into active signaling molecules. This creates a system where structure determines signaling capacity. When lipid composition is stable and substrates are available in the correct proportions, signaling proceeds with precision. When it is not, the signals themselves become inconsistent.

Cell membranes act as the platform where many of these signals originate. The arrangement of lipids within the membrane determines how receptors function, how enzymes are positioned, and how quickly signaling molecules can be generated and released. Membrane fluidity and organization influence the interaction between signaling proteins and their lipid environment. When membrane composition supports these interactions, signals are generated and transmitted efficiently. When it does not, receptor activity and downstream signaling pathways become less reliable.

Many signaling molecules are derived directly from membrane lipids. Enzymatic activity releases specific fatty acid components that are then converted into active mediators. These molecules act locally, altering cellular behavior in response to changes in the environment. The availability of these substrates depends on both dietary input and the efficiency of lipid digestion and transport. When the supply of lipid substrates is consistent, signaling output remains stable. When it fluctuates, the production of signaling molecules varies accordingly.

The timing of lipid-based signaling reflects changes in substrate availability and cellular demand. Signals can be generated rapidly in response to stimuli, but their magnitude depends on the pool of available lipid components. When these pools are maintained through consistent digestion and transport, signaling responses remain proportional to the stimulus. When substrate availability is limited or uneven, signaling may be reduced or delayed, affecting how cells respond to changes in their environment.

Lipid transport systems also influence signaling by determining how substrates are distributed across tissues. Lipoproteins deliver fatty acids and cholesterol to different regions of the body, affecting the composition of local membranes and the availability of signaling precursors. This distribution creates variation in signaling capacity between tissues, reflecting both their function and their access to lipid substrates. When transport is aligned, these differences support specialized functions. When it is not, signaling capacity may be reduced in some areas while remaining intact in others.

The interaction between lipid digestion, transport, and signaling creates a continuous chain that links dietary input to cellular response. Digestion determines which substrates are available, transport distributes them, and membrane organization converts them into signals. Disruption at any stage alters the entire system, changing both the availability of signaling molecules and the conditions under which they are generated.

Lipid-based signaling systems therefore depend on structural integrity and substrate availability. They are not independent pathways but extensions of membrane architecture and lipid metabolism. When these underlying systems are aligned, signaling remains consistent and responsive. When they are not, the generation and transmission of signals reflect the same variability, influencing how cells and tissues coordinate their activity.

Transport as Regulation

Transport is not a passive step that follows digestion. It functions as a control layer that determines how quickly nutrients appear in circulation, which tissues receive them, and in what form they arrive. The structure of transport particles, the pathways they move through, and the signals that govern their clearance define the rate and pattern of nutrient delivery. This means regulation is embedded in movement itself. Changing how a nutrient is transported changes how it is used.

Lipid transport illustrates this directly. After absorption, fatty acids are repackaged into chylomicrons that enter the lymphatic system before reaching the bloodstream. This routing delays their appearance in circulation and spreads delivery over time. The size and composition of these particles determine how they interact with tissues and enzymes that release fatty acids. Larger particles persist longer and deliver lipids gradually, while smaller or rapidly cleared particles shift delivery toward specific tissues more quickly. The transport structure sets the tempo of availability.

Enzymes that act on transport particles add another layer of control. As chylomicrons circulate, their contents are released in response to tissue demand and hormonal signals. This release is not uniform across the body. Some tissues increase extraction under certain conditions, while others reduce it, creating a distribution pattern that reflects current needs. The same amount of lipid can be directed toward storage or toward immediate use depending on how these transport interactions are regulated. Movement through the system becomes a mechanism for allocation.

Water-soluble nutrients follow a faster route through the bloodstream, but their transport is still regulated by carrier systems and concentration gradients. Rapid entry into circulation increases availability, but uptake into tissues depends on transport proteins and signaling states that control entry into cells. When transport into tissues is limited, these nutrients remain in circulation longer or are redirected toward storage pathways. The speed of transport therefore influences both availability and fate.

The timing of transport also determines how nutrients interact with one another. Lipids delivered through chylomicrons arrive over an extended period, while glucose and amino acids appear more rapidly. This difference creates a sequence of availability that affects how the body processes each substrate. When these timelines are aligned, energy use and storage remain coordinated. When they are not, nutrients compete or are redirected, altering the overall pattern of metabolism.

Transport pathways also influence where regulation occurs. Lipids passing through the lymphatic system bypass immediate hepatic processing, allowing peripheral tissues to receive them first. Water-soluble nutrients pass directly to the liver, where their distribution is modified before reaching the rest of the body. These route differences create distinct regulatory points that shape how nutrients are handled after absorption.

Transport therefore acts as a regulatory system by controlling timing, distribution, and interaction between nutrients. It determines whether substrates are delivered in a steady flow or in rapid pulses, whether they are directed toward specific tissues or dispersed broadly, and whether they are used immediately or stored. The structure and behavior of transport systems define how digestion translates into physiological outcome, making movement itself a primary mechanism of control.

PART VII

THE MICROBIOME AS A RESPONSE SYSTEM

Chapter 15

Microbial Behavior as a Digestive Output

Microbial behavior in the gut reflects the condition of digestion rather than acting as an independent driver of symptoms. The microbial population responds to the substrates that reach it, and those substrates are determined by how effectively upstream processes reduce and absorb nutrients. When digestion proceeds in sequence, most proteins, fats, and carbohydrates are processed into absorbable forms before reaching the distal intestine. The microbial environment then operates on a limited and consistent substrate pool. When digestion is incomplete, larger fragments and unprocessed nutrients move downstream, expanding the available substrate and altering microbial activity.

The composition of luminal contents defines microbial behavior. Bacteria metabolize what is present, not what was consumed. When proteins are fully reduced and absorbed, minimal protein substrate reaches the colon. When breakdown is incomplete, larger peptides and amino acids persist, providing material for microbial metabolism. The same applies to carbohydrates and fats. Undigested carbohydrates increase fermentable substrate, while improperly processed fats alter the physical environment in which microbes operate. The microbial response follows these changes directly.

Fermentation is the primary expression of this response. When fermentable substrates increase, microbial activity accelerates, producing gases and metabolic byproducts that change the internal environment. This affects motility, pressure within the intestine, and the chemical composition of luminal contents. The system reacts to these changes through adjustments in transit speed and secretion, but these responses are driven by the altered substrate conditions created upstream.

The distribution of substrates also influences where microbial activity is concentrated. When digestion is aligned, most substrates are absorbed earlier in the small intestine, and microbial activity remains more distal. When processing is incomplete, substrates appear earlier and in greater amounts, shifting microbial activity proximally. This changes the pattern of fermentation and alters how the intestine experiences and responds to microbial metabolism.

Microbial populations adapt to the substrates they encounter. A consistent input produces a stable microbial pattern, while variability in substrate delivery leads to shifts in population behavior. These shifts are not random. They reflect changes in nutrient availability and the physical environment within the gut. When upstream digestion is stable, microbial activity remains predictable. When it is not, microbial behavior fluctuates in response to changing conditions.

Immune interaction with the microbial environment is also influenced by digestion. The intestinal barrier is exposed to both microbial products and residual dietary substrates. When digestion is complete, exposure to larger, reactive molecules is limited. When it is not, these molecules interact with the epithelial surface alongside microbial byproducts, increasing signaling within the immune system. This interaction reflects the combined effect of digestion and microbial metabolism rather than the action of microbes alone.

Microbial behavior therefore represents an output of the digestive system. It is shaped by the substrates delivered to it, the timing of that delivery, and the physical conditions within the intestine. When digestion is aligned, microbial activity operates within a stable framework. When it is not, microbial behavior shifts in response to increased and variable substrate availability, and these changes propagate through the rest of the digestive system.

Fermentation from Incomplete Digestion

Fermentation increases when substrates that should have been reduced and absorbed earlier in the sequence reach regions of the intestine where microbial populations are prepared to metabolize them. This is not a random occurrence. It reflects a failure of upstream processing to convert macronutrients into absorbable forms. When proteins, carbohydrates, or fats remain partially intact, they become available to microbes as alternative substrates. The intensity and location of fermentation are determined by how much of this material escapes earlier stages and where it accumulates.

Carbohydrates are the most immediate driver of fermentation because they can be rapidly metabolized when they are not fully reduced to simple sugars and absorbed. Larger carbohydrate fragments that persist in the lumen provide a continuous substrate for microbial activity. As these molecules are metabolized, gases and byproducts are generated, altering the internal environment. This change affects motility and pressure, creating a feedback loop where the system adjusts transit speed in response to the altered conditions.

Protein fermentation follows a similar pattern but reflects a different type of upstream failure. When gastric and enzymatic processing do not fully reduce proteins to small peptides and amino acids, larger fragments remain available for microbial metabolism. These substrates are processed into compounds that change the chemical environment within the intestine. The presence of these compounds influences how the intestinal lining responds and how motility is regulated, contributing to variability in digestive behavior.

Fat contributes indirectly to fermentation when its digestion is impaired. Poor emulsification and incomplete breakdown leave lipids in forms that alter the physical environment of the intestine. This can change how carbohydrates and proteins are processed and how substrates are distributed within the lumen. As a result, fermentation patterns shift, not because fats themselves are rapidly fermented, but because they influence the availability and distribution of other substrates.

The location of fermentation reflects where substrates first exceed absorptive capacity. When digestion is aligned, most substrates are absorbed before reaching regions with dense microbial populations, and fermentation remains limited and distal. When upstream processing is incomplete, substrates appear earlier and in greater amounts, shifting fermentation proximally. This change increases the interaction between microbial activity and the upper sections of the intestine, where the system is less adapted to handle large amounts of fermentation.

The consequences of increased fermentation extend beyond gas production. The byproducts of microbial metabolism alter the luminal environment, affecting pH, motility, and epithelial interaction. These changes influence how the intestine processes subsequent substrates, creating a cycle where incomplete digestion leads to fermentation, which then alters the conditions for further digestion.

Fermentation from incomplete digestion therefore represents a downstream expression of upstream failure. It reflects the presence of substrates that were not reduced and absorbed in sequence. The intensity, location, and effects of fermentation are determined by how much of this material escapes earlier stages and how it interacts with the microbial environment that receives it.

Substrate Overload and Gas Production

Gas production increases when the amount of undigested substrate entering a region of the intestine exceeds the local capacity for absorption and controlled processing. This condition develops when upstream stages fail to reduce macronutrients into transportable forms, allowing larger fragments of carbohydrates and proteins to persist in the lumen. These fragments accumulate and become available to microbial populations that rapidly metabolize them. The result is not simply the presence of gas, but a shift in how the intestinal environment handles incoming material, driven by excess substrate rather than normal digestive flow.

The threshold for overload is determined by the balance between delivery and processing capacity. When gastric emptying is regulated and enzymatic activity is aligned with substrate arrival, nutrients are reduced and absorbed before they accumulate. When this balance is disrupted, larger amounts of partially processed material enter the intestine in a shorter time frame. Enzymes cannot keep pace with the incoming load, and transport systems cannot absorb substrates quickly enough to clear them. The excess remains in the lumen, where microbial metabolism becomes the dominant pathway for its breakdown.

Carbohydrates are the primary contributors to rapid gas production under these conditions because they are readily metabolized by microbes when not fully reduced to absorbable sugars. As microbial activity increases, gases are generated as byproducts of substrate breakdown. The rate of gas production reflects both the amount of substrate available and the speed at which microbes can process it. When substrate load is high, gas production rises quickly, increasing luminal pressure and altering the mechanical state of the intestine.

Protein contributes to gas production when it is not fully reduced and absorbed earlier in the sequence. Larger peptide fragments that reach the distal intestine provide additional substrate for microbial metabolism, generating a different profile of byproducts that further alter the luminal environment. These compounds influence motility and epithelial interaction, compounding the effects of carbohydrate-driven fermentation and contributing to variability in digestive behavior.

Fat influences substrate overload indirectly by shaping the conditions under which other macronutrients are processed. When lipid digestion is aligned, it slows gastric emptying and distributes substrate delivery over time, preventing sudden increases in load. When fat processing is impaired, this pacing function is reduced, and larger amounts of partially processed material can enter the intestine more rapidly. This accelerates the transition from manageable substrate levels to overload, increasing the likelihood of fermentation-driven gas production.

The mechanical effects of gas accumulation feed back into the digestive sequence. Increased pressure within the lumen alters motility patterns, changing how contents move and how long they remain in contact with absorptive surfaces. These changes can further reduce processing efficiency, allowing additional substrate to persist and reinforcing the cycle of overload and fermentation.

Substrate overload and gas production therefore represent a quantitative failure within the digestive sequence. When the amount of unprocessed material exceeds the capacity of enzymatic and absorptive systems, microbial metabolism becomes the dominant pathway for its breakdown. The resulting gas production reflects this shift and contributes to changes in the physical and functional state of the intestine.

Microbiome Shaped by Digestion, Not Vice Versa

The microbiome reflects the output of digestion rather than acting as the primary driver of digestive function. Microbial populations adapt to the substrates that reach them, and those substrates are determined by how effectively upstream processes reduce and absorb nutrients. When digestion proceeds in sequence, most macronutrients are processed and absorbed before they enter regions of dense microbial activity. The remaining substrate is limited and consistent, and microbial behavior stabilizes around that input. When digestion is incomplete, larger amounts of partially processed material move downstream, expanding the substrate pool and shifting microbial activity.

The type and quantity of substrate define microbial composition. Bacteria metabolize what is available in the lumen, not what is consumed at the level of the diet. When proteins are fully reduced and absorbed, minimal protein substrate reaches the colon. When this reduction is incomplete, larger fragments persist and become available for microbial metabolism. The same pattern applies to carbohydrates and fats. Increased delivery of fermentable substrates drives changes in microbial activity, which then alters the chemical and physical environment of the intestine.

These changes in microbial behavior are secondary to the conditions established earlier in the digestive sequence. Fermentation, gas production, and the generation of metabolic byproducts increase when substrate availability rises. These outputs influence motility, luminal pressure, and epithelial interaction, but they do not originate independently. They reflect the presence of substrates that were not processed upstream. The microbiome responds to these conditions, amplifying their effects within the intestine.

The location of microbial activity also shifts with changes in digestion. When upstream processing is effective, most substrates are absorbed before reaching distal regions, and microbial metabolism remains localized. When digestion is impaired, substrates appear earlier and in greater amounts, moving microbial activity proximally. This alters the pattern of fermentation and increases interaction between microbial byproducts and the upper sections of the intestine.

Microbial populations adapt over time to the substrate patterns they encounter. A stable digestive sequence produces a stable microbial environment. Variability in digestion produces variability in substrate delivery, leading to shifts in microbial composition and behavior. These shifts are not independent drivers but reflections of changing conditions within the lumen.

Understanding the microbiome as a downstream output clarifies the relationship between digestion and microbial activity. Interventions that focus solely on altering microbial populations without addressing upstream digestion do not change the underlying substrate conditions that drive microbial behavior. Restoring digestive sequence reduces the delivery of unprocessed material, stabilizing the environment in which microbes operate and allowing microbial patterns to normalize in response to consistent input.

Chapter 16

Dysbiosis as a Secondary Effect

Dysbiosis develops when the substrate environment within the intestine changes, not as an isolated event but as a downstream consequence of disrupted digestion. Microbial populations reorganize in response to what reaches them, and that input is determined by how effectively upstream processes reduce and absorb nutrients. When digestion proceeds in sequence, the majority of macronutrients are processed and absorbed before entering regions of dense microbial activity, and the remaining substrate supports a stable microbial pattern. When this sequence breaks, larger quantities of partially processed material move downstream, altering the conditions that shape microbial behavior.

The defining feature of dysbiosis is a shift in substrate availability. Increased delivery of fermentable carbohydrates, undigested proteins, or improperly processed fats expands the energy sources available to microbes. This changes the balance of microbial activity, favoring organisms that can metabolize these substrates under the new conditions. The shift is not random. It reflects the composition and distribution of the material entering the microbial environment. As substrate patterns change, microbial populations adjust accordingly.

This adjustment affects the chemical and physical environment within the intestine. As microbial metabolism increases, the production of gases and metabolic byproducts rises, altering luminal pressure, pH, and motility patterns. These changes feed back into the digestive sequence, influencing how contents move and how subsequent substrates are processed. The system responds to these altered conditions, but the response is reactive and does not restore the original coordination of digestion.

The location of dysbiotic activity also reflects upstream failure. When digestion is aligned, microbial metabolism is largely confined to distal regions where substrate availability is lower and more consistent. When digestion is impaired, substrates appear earlier in the intestine, shifting microbial activity proximally. This change increases the interaction between microbial byproducts and the intestinal lining in regions that are not adapted to high levels of fermentation, amplifying the effects on motility and signaling.

Immune interaction follows the same pattern. Increased exposure to microbial byproducts and partially digested substrates alters signaling at the epithelial surface. This interaction reflects the combined effect of digestion and microbial metabolism rather than the action of microbes alone. The immune system responds to the environment it encounters, which is shaped by both substrate composition and microbial activity.

Dysbiosis therefore represents a secondary effect of changes in the digestive sequence. It is the outcome of altered substrate delivery, distribution, and processing rather than an independent cause of dysfunction. Addressing dysbiosis requires understanding the upstream conditions that produce the substrate patterns driving microbial behavior. When digestion is restored and substrate delivery returns to a stable pattern, microbial populations adjust in response to the new environment, and dysbiotic patterns resolve as a consequence of that change.

Microbial Imbalance as Downstream Consequence

Microbial imbalance develops when the substrate landscape within the intestine changes, and that landscape is set by digestion. The microbiome does not select its inputs. It metabolizes what arrives. When upstream processes reduce proteins, carbohydrates, and fats into absorbable forms and move them across the epithelial barrier in sequence, only a limited and predictable amount of substrate reaches the distal gut. Under those conditions, microbial activity stabilizes because its fuel supply is consistent in both quantity and composition. When digestion fails to complete that reduction, larger fragments persist and pass forward, expanding the substrate pool and shifting microbial behavior in direct proportion to that change.

The character of the imbalance reflects the type of substrate that escapes absorption. Excess carbohydrate fragments increase rapid fermentation and gas generation because they are readily metabolized. Incomplete protein breakdown introduces larger peptides and amino acids that are processed along different metabolic routes, changing the chemical profile of the lumen. Impaired fat digestion alters dispersion and mixing, changing how substrates are distributed and how microbes access them. These are not independent microbial decisions. They are responses to the material present. As substrate patterns change, microbial populations reorganize to match the available energy sources.

Location follows the same logic. When digestion is aligned, most substrates are absorbed proximally, and microbial activity remains concentrated distally. When processing is incomplete, substrates appear earlier in the intestine, shifting microbial metabolism toward regions that are not designed to handle high levels of fermentation. This increases local gas production and changes motility patterns in those segments. The intestine responds to pressure and chemical changes by altering transit, but those adjustments are reactions to a substrate condition that originated upstream.

The physical environment reinforces the imbalance. Accumulated substrates increase luminal density and create uneven distribution, producing regions of high and low activity within the same segment. This heterogeneity affects how contents mix and how long they remain in contact with the epithelial surface. Areas with concentrated substrate drive intense microbial metabolism, while adjacent areas process less. The result is variability in fermentation, pressure, and chemical output across short distances, which further disrupts coordinated motility.

Immune signaling tracks these changes because the epithelial surface encounters both microbial products and residual dietary fragments at the same time. When digestion is complete, exposure is limited to defined molecular forms and controlled microbial byproducts. When it is not, larger fragments and increased microbial metabolites interact with the barrier together, increasing signaling intensity. The response reflects the combined environment rather than a single microbial factor.

Microbial imbalance is therefore a downstream consequence of altered substrate delivery and distribution. It arises when digestion fails to constrain what reaches the microbial environment, allowing quantity, form, and location of substrates to shift. The resulting changes in microbial behavior, gas production, and chemical output are expressions of that upstream failure. Restoring balance requires restoring the sequence that limits and defines the substrate entering the system, because the microbiome will always reorganize around the inputs it receives.

Why Treating Microbes Alone Fails

Interventions that target microbes without changing digestion leave the underlying substrate conditions untouched, so the microbial pattern returns to its prior state once the intervention is removed. The microbiome is shaped by the material that reaches it. If partially digested proteins, carbohydrates, and fats continue to enter the distal intestine, microbes will reorganize around those inputs regardless of how often the population is suppressed or modified. The system resets to match the available fuel. Removing organisms does not remove the conditions that select for them.

The limitation becomes clear when considering how substrates arrive in the microbial environment. Upstream digestion determines whether nutrients are reduced and absorbed or whether they persist in larger fragments. When this reduction is incomplete, the lumen carries an expanded and variable substrate load into regions where microbial metabolism dominates. Any attempt to alter microbial composition without reducing this load addresses the response rather than the cause. The same substrates remain available, and microbial populations that can utilize them reestablish.

Timing and distribution reinforce this pattern. When gastric emptying is irregular or when enzymatic activity is misaligned with substrate arrival, nutrients reach the intestine in pulses that exceed local capacity. These pulses create transient conditions of overload that favor rapid microbial metabolism. Even if microbial populations are temporarily reduced, the repeated delivery of excess substrate recreates the same environment, and the system returns to the same state. The sequence of digestion continues to produce the conditions that drive microbial behavior.

The physical environment within the intestine also remains unchanged when digestion is not corrected. Poor emulsification, uneven substrate distribution, and altered motility patterns create regions where microbial activity is concentrated. These structural conditions persist regardless of interventions aimed at the microbes themselves. As long as the environment supports uneven processing and localized substrate accumulation, microbial patterns will reflect that structure.

Immune interaction follows the same dependency. Increased exposure to microbial byproducts and partially digested substrates results from the combined effect of digestion and microbial metabolism. Targeting microbes alone does not reduce the presence of these substrates, so the signals generated at the epithelial surface remain elevated. The system continues to respond to the same inputs, maintaining the conditions that support imbalance.

Treating microbes alone fails because it does not change the sequence that delivers substrates into the microbial environment. Digestion defines what reaches the microbes, how much of it arrives, and where it accumulates. Without correcting these upstream processes, interventions aimed at microbial populations operate against a system that continues to produce the same inputs. The microbiome will reorganize around those inputs as long as they persist, making lasting change dependent on restoring the digestive sequence that limits and defines substrate delivery.

PART VIII

IMMUNE SYSTEM AND DIGESTION

Chapter 17

Immune Activation in the Gut

Immune activation in the gut reflects the condition of the material presented to the intestinal barrier rather than an isolated malfunction of the immune system itself. The epithelial surface is continuously exposed to both dietary substrates and microbial byproducts, and the form in which these arrive determines the level of immune signaling that is generated. When digestion proceeds in sequence, most nutrients are reduced to defined molecular units and absorbed before reaching the distal intestine. The barrier encounters a controlled set of inputs, and immune activity remains within a stable range. When digestion is incomplete, larger fragments and increased microbial metabolites reach the epithelial surface together, amplifying signaling within the system.

The structure of the substrate is the first determinant of immune interaction. Small peptides, amino acids, and simple sugars interact with the epithelial surface in a predictable manner and are rapidly transported across the membrane. Larger fragments persist in the lumen and increase contact with the barrier. This prolonged interaction changes how the epithelial layer responds, increasing signaling intensity and altering the local environment. The difference lies in the form of the substrate rather than its identity.

Microbial activity compounds this effect by generating additional compounds from the substrates that reach it. When fermentation increases due to incomplete digestion, microbial byproducts accumulate and interact with the epithelial surface alongside residual dietary fragments. This combination changes the chemical conditions within the lumen and increases the complexity of signals encountered by the barrier. The immune system responds to this combined environment, integrating signals from both microbial metabolism and unprocessed substrates.

The location of these interactions influences their impact. When digestion is aligned, most substrate exposure occurs in distal regions where the system is adapted to handle microbial activity. When upstream processing fails, substrates appear earlier in the intestine, shifting immune interaction proximally. This increases exposure in regions where the barrier is not adapted to sustained contact with large amounts of microbial byproducts and partially digested material, amplifying the response.

Motility and luminal pressure also contribute to immune activation by altering the duration and intensity of exposure. Increased gas production and irregular transit patterns change how long substrates remain in contact with the epithelial surface. Prolonged retention increases the opportunity for interaction, while rapid transit can deliver substrates in forms that have not been fully processed. Both conditions reflect upstream variability and influence the level of immune signaling generated.

Immune activation therefore represents an output of the digestive sequence, shaped by the structure, quantity, and distribution of substrates within the intestine. It arises when the barrier is exposed to material that has not been reduced and absorbed in sequence, combined with increased microbial byproducts generated from that material. The response reflects the environment created by digestion and microbial activity rather than an independent failure of the immune system.

Exposure to Incomplete Food Fragments

Exposure to incomplete food fragments occurs when upstream digestion fails to reduce macronutrients into the molecular forms required for membrane transport. Proteins that should be converted into small peptides and amino acids, carbohydrates that should be reduced to simple sugars, and lipids that should be dispersed and cleaved into transportable units remain partially intact. These larger fragments persist within the lumen and increase contact with the intestinal barrier. The epithelial surface is then presented with material that extends beyond its normal handling range, changing the nature and intensity of local signaling.

The duration of exposure is determined by motility and the physical state of luminal contents. When digestion is aligned, substrates are reduced and absorbed quickly, limiting the time they remain in contact with the epithelial surface. When reduction is incomplete, these fragments remain within the lumen for longer periods, increasing the opportunity for interaction. Irregular motility further alters this exposure by either prolonging retention or delivering partially processed material more rapidly into downstream regions. In both cases, the barrier encounters substrates that have not been prepared for immediate uptake.

The structural properties of these fragments influence how they interact with the epithelial layer. Larger molecules present more complex surfaces and persist at the interface between the lumen and the membrane, altering how transport systems and surface receptors engage with them. This changes the pattern of signaling within the epithelial cells, increasing activity in pathways that respond to luminal content. The response is driven by the form and persistence of the substrate rather than by its origin.

Microbial metabolism amplifies this exposure by acting on the same incomplete fragments. As microbes process these substrates, they generate additional compounds that accumulate alongside the original material. This creates a combined environment where dietary fragments and microbial byproducts interact with the epithelial surface simultaneously. The barrier responds to the totality of this environment, integrating signals from both sources.

The location of exposure shifts when upstream digestion is impaired. Instead of being confined to distal regions, incomplete fragments appear earlier in the intestine, increasing contact with sections that are not adapted to sustained exposure. This alters the distribution of interaction along the digestive tract and changes how different regions respond to luminal content.

Exposure to incomplete food fragments therefore reflects a failure of the digestive sequence to produce absorbable forms. It increases both the duration and complexity of interaction at the epithelial surface, altering signaling within the intestinal barrier. The extent of this exposure is determined by how much material escapes upstream processing, how long it remains in the lumen, and where it accumulates within the digestive tract.

Barrier Stress and Immune Signaling

Barrier stress develops when the epithelial surface is exposed to substrates and byproducts that exceed its normal processing range, and immune signaling increases as a direct response to that exposure. The intestinal barrier is designed to interface with defined molecular forms that can be transported across the membrane or cleared efficiently. When digestion proceeds in sequence, most substrates are reduced to these forms before reaching the epithelial surface, and contact remains controlled. When upstream processing fails, larger fragments and increased microbial metabolites persist in the lumen, extending both the duration and intensity of contact with the barrier.

The physical state of luminal contents determines how this stress develops. Poorly reduced substrates remain in larger, more complex forms that interact with the epithelial surface over a wider area and for longer periods. These fragments alter the local environment at the membrane interface, changing how epithelial cells respond to what they encounter. Instead of rapid transport and clearance, the system shifts toward increased signaling, reflecting the presence of material that cannot be processed through standard pathways.

Microbial metabolism amplifies barrier stress by generating additional compounds from the same substrates. As fermentation increases, these byproducts accumulate alongside partially digested material, creating a combined environment that differs from the conditions present during coordinated digestion. The epithelial surface responds to both sources simultaneously, and the signaling intensity reflects the total burden of luminal content rather than a single input.

Motility and pressure further influence this interaction. Increased gas production and irregular transit patterns change how long substrates remain in contact with the epithelial surface and how they are distributed along the intestine. Prolonged retention increases exposure time, while uneven distribution creates localized regions of higher stress. These mechanical and temporal factors contribute to variability in how the barrier experiences luminal content.

The location of barrier stress shifts when digestion is impaired. Instead of being concentrated in distal regions, exposure to complex substrates and microbial byproducts occurs earlier in the intestine. This increases interaction in regions that are not adapted to sustained exposure, amplifying the signaling response and altering how the barrier functions in those areas.

Barrier stress and immune signaling therefore arise from the interaction between incomplete digestion and microbial metabolism. They reflect the condition of the luminal environment rather than an isolated immune process. When digestion is aligned, exposure remains limited and signaling stays within a stable range. When it is not, increased and prolonged contact with complex substrates and byproducts drives a higher level of immune activity as the system responds to the environment it encounters.

Chapter 18

Food Sensitivity as a Digestive Failure

Food sensitivity emerges when the digestive system fails to convert incoming food into forms that can be absorbed without extended interaction with the intestinal barrier. The reaction is not defined by the food itself but by the condition in which that food reaches the epithelial surface. When digestion proceeds in sequence, proteins are reduced to small peptides and amino acids, carbohydrates to simple sugars, and fats to dispersed, transportable structures. These forms move across the membrane quickly, limiting exposure. When this sequence breaks, larger fragments persist in the lumen, increasing both the duration and complexity of contact with the barrier and shifting the system toward reactivity.

The variability of food sensitivity reflects the variability of digestion. The same food can be tolerated under conditions where gastric processing, enzyme activity, and bile flow are aligned, and can provoke symptoms when those conditions are disrupted. This inconsistency is a direct result of how substrates are presented to the intestine. When proteins are not fully unfolded and cleaved, larger fragments remain available to interact with the epithelial surface. When carbohydrates are not fully reduced, they persist and contribute to fermentation. When fats are not properly emulsified, they alter the physical environment and delay the coordinated processing of other nutrients. Each of these failures increases the likelihood of prolonged exposure.

The sequence of digestion determines whether these fragments are cleared or retained. Gastric acid sets the structural state of proteins, pancreatic enzymes complete their reduction, and bile organizes lipids into forms that support efficient breakdown and absorption. When any part of this sequence is weakened or mistimed, substrates move forward in incomplete forms. These forms do not engage transport systems effectively, so they remain within the lumen and increase contact with the epithelial surface. The response that follows is driven by this exposure rather than by an inherent property of the food.

Microbial activity amplifies this effect by acting on the same incomplete substrates. As fermentation increases, microbial byproducts accumulate alongside dietary fragments, altering the luminal environment and increasing signaling at the epithelial interface. This combined exposure changes how the intestine responds to subsequent inputs, reinforcing a pattern where sensitivity becomes more likely as digestion remains misaligned.

Motility and timing contribute to the persistence of this state. Irregular gastric emptying and altered intestinal transit change how long substrates remain in contact with the epithelial surface and where that contact occurs. Prolonged retention increases exposure, while rapid transit can deliver partially processed material into regions not prepared to handle it. Both conditions reflect upstream disruption and contribute to variability in response.

Food sensitivity therefore represents a failure of the digestive sequence to produce absorbable forms and clear them efficiently. It arises when substrates remain in the lumen long enough and in forms complex enough to alter interaction with the intestinal barrier. The specific foods associated with symptoms reflect the conditions under which they are processed rather than fixed properties of those foods. Restoring sequence reduces exposure, allowing the same foods to be handled without triggering the responses that define sensitivity.

Immune Response to Poor Processing

The immune response in the gut increases when digestion fails to convert food into forms that can be rapidly transported across the epithelial barrier. The system is built to encounter defined molecular units that pass through the membrane with minimal interaction. When proteins remain as larger fragments, when carbohydrates are not fully reduced, or when lipids are not properly dispersed, these substrates persist in the lumen and extend their contact with the epithelial surface. The immune response reflects this prolonged and altered exposure rather than the presence of the food itself.

The structure of the substrate determines how the barrier interprets it. Small molecules move through transport systems with limited engagement, while larger fragments remain at the interface between the lumen and the membrane. This persistence increases the probability of interaction with epithelial cells and the signaling pathways they control. The response is driven by the form and duration of contact. As the size and complexity of the substrate increase, so does the level of signaling generated at the barrier.

Microbial metabolism amplifies this process by acting on the same incompletely digested material. As microbes break down these substrates, they produce additional compounds that accumulate alongside the original fragments. The epithelial surface is then exposed to a combined environment of dietary and microbial products. This mixture changes the chemical conditions within the lumen and increases the complexity of signals encountered by the barrier. The immune response reflects the total environment rather than a single source.

Timing and motility shape how this interaction unfolds. When digestion is aligned, substrates are cleared quickly, and exposure remains brief. When processing is incomplete, fragments remain in contact with the epithelial surface for longer periods. Irregular motility can further increase exposure by prolonging retention or by delivering partially processed material into regions where it would not normally appear. These changes alter both the duration and location of interaction, influencing the level of immune signaling.

The location of exposure is critical because different regions of the intestine are adapted to different levels of substrate and microbial contact. When digestion is functioning properly, most interaction with complex substrates occurs distally. When it is not, these substrates appear earlier in the intestine, increasing immune activity in regions that are not designed to handle sustained exposure. This shift amplifies the response and contributes to variability in how the system reacts to incoming food.

The immune response to poor processing therefore reflects a mismatch between substrate form and the conditions required for efficient absorption. It arises when digestion fails to complete its sequence, leaving larger and more complex material in contact with the epithelial surface. The resulting signaling is a direct consequence of that exposure, shaped by the structure, quantity, and distribution of substrates within the intestine.

Loss of Tolerance as System Instability

Loss of tolerance develops when the digestive system stops producing consistent substrate conditions and begins delivering variable inputs to the intestinal barrier. Tolerance depends on predictability. When proteins are reduced to the same small forms, when carbohydrates arrive as simple sugars, and when lipids are dispersed and matched with bile and enzymes, the epithelial surface encounters a stable pattern of substrates. Under these conditions, transport proceeds quickly and interaction remains brief. When this consistency breaks, the system is exposed to a shifting range of fragment sizes, concentrations, and delivery rates, and tolerance narrows as a result.

Instability begins with disruption in sequence. Variations in gastric acid output, enzyme activity, bile flow, and motility change how food is processed from one meal to the next. The same food can be reduced efficiently under one set of conditions and remain partially intact under another. This inconsistency alters the form of the substrate presented to the intestine. Larger fragments persist during periods of reduced processing, increasing exposure to the epithelial surface and amplifying signaling. Over time, this repeated variability changes how the system responds, making it more likely to react even when conditions temporarily improve.

The distribution of substrates contributes to this instability. When digestion is aligned, nutrients are delivered and absorbed in a steady flow. When it is not, substrates arrive in uneven pulses or remain in the lumen longer than expected. These fluctuations create alternating periods of low and high exposure, preventing the system from maintaining a stable interaction pattern. The barrier adapts to this variability by increasing sensitivity to changes in substrate presence, further reducing tolerance.

Microbial activity reinforces this pattern. As incomplete substrates reach the distal intestine, fermentation increases and generates additional byproducts that alter the luminal environment. These changes feed back into the system, affecting motility and the conditions under which subsequent meals are processed. The result is a cycle where variability in digestion leads to variability in microbial output, which then increases variability in the digestive environment itself.

The immune response tracks this instability. As the epithelial surface encounters a wider range of substrate forms and microbial byproducts, signaling becomes less predictable and more reactive. The system no longer operates within a narrow range of expected inputs. Instead, it responds to a fluctuating environment where the same food may produce different substrate conditions depending on the state of digestion at that time.

Loss of tolerance therefore reflects a system that has lost its ability to maintain consistent processing and delivery of nutrients. It is not tied to a specific food but to the variability in how that food is handled. When the digestive sequence is restored and substrate delivery becomes consistent again, the conditions that drive instability are reduced, and tolerance can return as the system reestablishes predictable interaction with incoming nutrients.

PART IX

SYSTEMIC EFFECTS OF DIGESTIVE FAILURE

Chapter 19

Energy and Metabolic Consequences

Energy production reflects how effectively the digestive system converts incoming food into substrates that can be absorbed, transported, and oxidized within cells. The sequence from digestion to cellular metabolism is continuous. When this sequence is aligned, nutrients are delivered in forms and at rates that match metabolic demand, allowing energy production to proceed with stability. When digestion is incomplete or irregular, the availability of substrates becomes inconsistent, and the entire metabolic system is forced to adjust to fluctuations in supply.

The first consequence appears in substrate availability. Proteins that are not fully reduced limit the pool of amino acids available for cellular processes. Carbohydrates that are not fully broken down reduce the supply of simple sugars that can be rapidly used for energy. Lipids that are not properly emulsified and absorbed limit the delivery of fatty acids that support sustained energy production. Each of these limitations reduces the total substrate pool available to cells, not because intake is low, but because delivery is incomplete.

Timing further shapes energy availability. When digestion and absorption are coordinated, nutrients enter circulation in a pattern that supports continuous metabolic activity. Water-soluble nutrients appear quickly, while lipid-derived substrates are delivered over a longer period through transport systems such as chylomicrons. This sequence provides both immediate and sustained energy sources. When digestion is disrupted, this timing becomes irregular. Substrates may arrive in pulses or in reduced amounts, creating periods where energy supply does not match demand.

Hormonal signaling responds to these changes in availability. When substrate delivery is consistent, hormonal signals align with metabolic needs, directing nutrients toward oxidation or storage in a coordinated manner. When delivery is inconsistent, signaling becomes reactive. Periods of reduced substrate availability are followed by periods of increased supply, and hormonal responses shift accordingly. This variability alters how nutrients are used, stored, and released, affecting overall metabolic stability.

The physical and chemical environment within the intestine also influences energy outcomes. Increased fermentation from incomplete digestion diverts substrates into microbial metabolism, reducing the amount available for absorption. The byproducts of this process alter the luminal environment and influence motility, further affecting how nutrients are processed and absorbed. The system loses efficiency as a portion of the energy contained in food is redirected away from the host.

At the cellular level, inconsistent substrate delivery affects how energy pathways operate. Cells rely on a steady supply of substrates to maintain stable production of energy. When supply fluctuates, cells adjust by altering substrate preference, shifting between available sources as conditions change. This adaptation maintains function but reduces efficiency and increases variability in output.

Energy and metabolic consequences therefore arise from how well the digestive sequence delivers substrates into the system. When digestion, absorption, and transport are aligned, energy production proceeds with consistency and efficiency. When they are not, substrate availability becomes irregular, hormonal signaling shifts, and cellular metabolism adapts to a variable supply. The outcome reflects the condition of the digestive system rather than the quantity of food consumed.

Incomplete Nutrient Extraction

Incomplete nutrient extraction occurs when the digestive system fails to convert ingested food into forms that can be absorbed and transported into the body. The quantity of food entering the system remains the same, but the fraction that becomes available to cells is reduced. This loss happens at the level of structure. Proteins that are not fully unfolded and cleaved, carbohydrates that are not reduced to simple sugars, and lipids that are not properly emulsified and broken down remain in the lumen and move forward without being captured by transport systems.

The limitation begins with preparation. Gastric acid sets the structural state of proteins, exposing sites where enzymes can act. When this step is incomplete, enzymatic access is restricted and larger fragments persist. Pancreatic enzymes depend on this prior reduction to complete breakdown. When substrate structure does not match enzymatic requirements, cleavage slows and a portion of the material remains outside the range that transport systems can handle. Lipids follow the same pattern. Without adequate emulsification, large fat aggregates limit enzyme contact and reduce the generation of absorbable components.

Transport systems enforce these structural requirements. The intestinal membrane accepts only defined molecular forms, and anything outside that range is excluded. Larger peptide fragments, partially reduced carbohydrates, and poorly organized lipid components do not cross into the body. They continue through the intestine, contributing to downstream processes such as fermentation rather than absorption. The presence of these nutrients within the lumen does not translate into availability within the system.

Timing and flow further influence extraction. When gastric emptying and intestinal motility are aligned, substrates are delivered in a steady pattern that allows enzymes and transporters to operate continuously. When delivery is irregular, substrates arrive in pulses that exceed local capacity. Enzymes cannot process the incoming load quickly enough, and transport systems cannot absorb it at the required rate. The excess remains in the lumen, reducing the proportion of nutrients that are captured.

The physical environment within the intestine also affects extraction efficiency. Uniform dispersion of substrates supports consistent enzymatic activity and absorption. When dispersion is incomplete, regions of high substrate concentration form, limiting enzyme access and creating uneven processing. These localized conditions reduce overall efficiency because portions of the substrate are not exposed to the conditions required for breakdown and uptake.

Incomplete nutrient extraction therefore reflects a failure of the digestive sequence to convert intake into usable output. It is not a matter of how much food is consumed but how much of that food is structurally prepared, processed, and transported into the body. When the sequence is aligned, extraction approaches the system's capacity. When it is not, a portion of the available nutrients remains outside the system, reducing the effective yield from the same intake.

Mitochondrial Energy Instability

Mitochondrial energy production depends on a continuous and properly structured supply of substrates delivered from digestion. When proteins, carbohydrates, and fats are reduced, absorbed, and transported in sequence, mitochondria receive a steady inflow of amino acids, glucose-derived intermediates, and fatty acids that can be oxidized in a coordinated manner. This continuity allows energy production to remain stable because substrate availability matches enzymatic capacity within the cell. When digestion is incomplete or irregular, that supply becomes inconsistent, and mitochondrial output reflects this variability.

The first disruption appears as fluctuation in substrate delivery. Incomplete digestion reduces the total amount of usable substrate entering circulation, while irregular gastric emptying and absorption create uneven timing. Mitochondria rely on a constant inflow of substrates to maintain stable energy production. When delivery occurs in pulses or in reduced amounts, cells must shift between available fuels, altering metabolic pathways to compensate for changing conditions. These shifts maintain function but reduce efficiency and introduce variability in energy output.

Lipid-derived substrates are central to maintaining stability because they provide a sustained source of energy when properly digested and transported. When fat digestion is aligned, fatty acids are delivered over an extended period through structured transport systems, supporting continuous mitochondrial activity. When lipid processing is impaired, this sustained supply is reduced, and the system becomes more dependent on rapidly fluctuating carbohydrate-derived substrates. This increases variability in energy production because these substrates are delivered more quickly and cleared more rapidly.

Hormonal signaling amplifies these effects by responding to changes in substrate availability. When nutrient delivery is stable, hormonal signals direct substrates into mitochondria in a coordinated manner. When delivery fluctuates, signaling becomes reactive, shifting between storage and utilization states. This alters how substrates are directed within the cell, affecting the balance between different energy pathways and contributing to instability in mitochondrial output.

The internal cellular environment also reflects these changes. Mitochondria operate within a network of enzymatic reactions that depend on the availability of substrates and cofactors. When substrate supply is inconsistent, these reactions cannot proceed at a steady rate. Intermediates accumulate or become depleted, altering the efficiency of energy production. The system adapts by adjusting pathway activity, but these adjustments introduce further variability.

Mitochondrial energy instability therefore arises from disruptions in the delivery of substrates from digestion through absorption and transport into the cell. It reflects a mismatch between the supply of usable nutrients and the requirements of cellular energy systems. When digestion and transport are aligned, substrate delivery supports consistent mitochondrial function. When they are not, fluctuations in availability force the system into continuous adjustment, reducing stability in energy production.

Chapter 20

Hormonal Instability

Hormonal stability depends on consistent substrate delivery, predictable transport patterns, and steady cellular conditions. When digestion, absorption, and lipid transport are aligned, nutrients enter circulation in a pattern that allows endocrine signaling to operate within a narrow and controlled range. Hormones respond to real conditions. When those conditions are stable, signaling remains proportional and coordinated. When digestion produces variable inputs, the signals that regulate metabolism, storage, and energy use begin to fluctuate because the system is reacting to an inconsistent environment.

The instability begins with irregular nutrient appearance in circulation. Carbohydrates that are not consistently reduced and absorbed produce variable glucose availability. Lipids that are not properly emulsified and transported reduce the steady delivery of fatty acids. Proteins that are incompletely processed limit the availability of amino acids that support structural and signaling pathways. These changes alter the signals that control how nutrients are handled. Hormonal responses shift to match what is present at that moment rather than following a predictable pattern.

Insulin reflects this variability directly. When glucose appears in a controlled and predictable manner, insulin release matches the rate of entry into circulation, directing substrates into tissues with precision. When glucose delivery is irregular, insulin output follows that variability, rising sharply during periods of rapid appearance and falling when supply declines. This creates alternating phases of storage and release that do not align with stable energy demand. The pattern reflects the inconsistency of substrate delivery rather than a primary defect in signaling.

Lipid-related signaling contributes to this instability when fat digestion is impaired. A consistent supply of fatty acids supports sustained energy use and moderates fluctuations in glucose handling. When lipid delivery is reduced or delayed, the system becomes more dependent on rapidly changing carbohydrate availability. Hormonal responses shift accordingly, increasing variability in how energy is allocated and used. The absence of steady lipid-derived substrates removes a stabilizing influence on the system.

Counter-regulatory hormones follow the same pattern. When substrate availability declines due to incomplete digestion or irregular absorption, signals that promote release of stored energy increase. When substrates appear again in higher amounts, signals shift back toward storage. This oscillation reflects the inconsistency of input rather than a coordinated response to stable demand. The system moves between opposing states because the conditions driving those states are not aligned.

The interaction between hormonal signaling and transport systems further shapes this instability. Transport determines how quickly nutrients appear in circulation and how they are distributed across tissues. When transport patterns are irregular, hormones must adjust to changes in both timing and location of substrate availability. This adds another layer of variability, as signaling responds not only to quantity but also to distribution.

Hormonal instability therefore reflects a system responding to inconsistent inputs generated by disrupted digestion and transport. It is not a primary failure of endocrine function but a consequence of variability in substrate availability and delivery. When digestion, absorption, and transport are aligned, hormonal signaling stabilizes because it is responding to predictable conditions. When they are not, signaling fluctuates as the system attempts to match an environment that is constantly changing.

Lipid Transport and Endocrine Signaling

Lipid transport defines how endocrine signals are generated, sustained, and resolved because it controls when fatty acids and cholesterol appear in circulation, how long they remain available, and which tissues receive them. After absorption, lipids are packaged into chylomicrons and routed through the lymphatic system before entering the bloodstream. This pathway delays their arrival and spreads delivery over time. The result is a prolonged, controlled input that shapes hormonal responses differently from the rapid appearance of water-soluble nutrients. Endocrine signaling follows this timing. When lipid delivery is steady, hormonal output remains proportional and sustained. When it is irregular, signaling becomes uneven because the substrate driving it is inconsistent.

The structure of transport particles determines how lipids interact with tissues and enzymes that release fatty acids. Chylomicrons carry triglycerides that are progressively hydrolyzed as they circulate, and this staged release creates a gradual supply of fatty acids to peripheral tissues. Hormonal signals regulate this process by altering how quickly these particles are processed and where their contents are delivered. When signals favor uptake, tissues extract fatty acids efficiently and circulating levels decline in a controlled manner. When signals reduce uptake, these particles persist longer, extending the availability of lipids in circulation. The interaction between transport structure and hormonal control sets the rate of delivery.

Cholesterol transport adds another dimension to this system because it provides the substrate for hormone synthesis. Lipoprotein particles deliver cholesterol to tissues that convert it into signaling molecules. The availability of cholesterol within these cells determines whether synthesis can proceed at a rate that matches demand. When lipid transport is consistent, cholesterol delivery supports stable hormone production. When transport is disrupted, the supply becomes uneven, and endocrine output reflects that limitation.

Lipid-derived signals also originate directly from transported substrates. Fatty acids and their derivatives influence how cells respond to incoming nutrients, altering pathways that control energy use, storage, and cellular behavior. The magnitude of these signals depends on the concentration and timing of lipid delivery. A steady influx produces a stable signaling environment. Fluctuations in delivery create variability in signal intensity, affecting how cells coordinate their responses.

The relationship between lipid transport and endocrine signaling becomes more apparent when compared to rapidly delivered substrates. Glucose enters circulation quickly and produces immediate hormonal responses that rise and fall over short periods. Lipids arrive more slowly and sustain signaling over longer intervals. When both systems are aligned, this combination provides both rapid and sustained control. When lipid transport is impaired, the system loses this sustained component and becomes dominated by faster, more variable signals.

Transport pathways also determine where endocrine signals are expressed. Lipids delivered through the lymphatic system reach peripheral tissues before passing through the liver, altering how signals are distributed across the body. This routing allows tissues outside the liver to respond directly to lipid availability. Changes in transport therefore shift not only the timing of signals but also their spatial distribution.

Lipid transport and endocrine signaling operate as a connected system where movement determines message. The rate, structure, and routing of lipid delivery define how hormonal signals are generated and maintained. When transport is aligned with digestion and tissue demand, signaling remains stable and coordinated. When it is not, variability in delivery produces variability in endocrine output, reflecting the same inconsistency present in the underlying substrate flow.

Stress Hormones and Digestive Suppression

Stress hormones shift the body into a state where immediate resource mobilization takes priority over processing incoming food. This shift alters blood flow, secretion patterns, and motility in ways that reduce digestive output at every stage. The stomach produces less acid, pancreatic enzyme release declines, bile flow becomes less coordinated, and intestinal movement changes in pattern and intensity. These changes are not isolated. They occur together as part of a coordinated response that reallocates energy and attention away from digestion and toward short-term demands.

The reduction in gastric acid changes the structural state of food entering the system. Proteins are not fully unfolded, limiting enzymatic access downstream. When this occurs, pancreatic enzymes receive substrates that do not match their requirements, and breakdown remains incomplete. Lipid processing is affected in parallel. Without proper coordination between gastric emptying and bile release, fats enter the intestine in forms that are not efficiently emulsified. This reduces the formation of absorbable lipid components and alters how other nutrients are processed in the same environment.

Pancreatic output depends on signals generated during early phases of digestion, and these signals are weakened when the system is under stress. Reduced enzyme release limits the system's ability to complete breakdown of proteins, carbohydrates, and fats. Substrates remain in larger forms and move forward in the sequence without being fully processed. This increases the amount of material that reaches distal regions of the intestine, where microbial metabolism becomes more prominent.

Motility patterns shift under stress as well. The coordinated movement that normally supports mixing and controlled progression becomes irregular. Some regions may move contents more rapidly, reducing contact time for enzymatic activity, while others may retain material longer, increasing exposure to partially processed substrates. This variability alters how substrates are distributed along the intestine and contributes to uneven processing.

Blood flow to the digestive tract decreases during stress, further limiting the system's capacity to produce secretions and maintain efficient absorption. Reduced perfusion affects the epithelial surface and the transport systems embedded within it, decreasing the rate at which nutrients can move into the body. This adds another layer of limitation, where even properly processed substrates may not be absorbed at full capacity.

The cumulative effect of these changes is a reduction in digestive efficiency that propagates through the entire sequence. Substrates are not prepared, not broken down, and not absorbed in alignment with the system's design. The result is increased delivery of incomplete material to downstream regions, altered microbial activity, and changes in the internal environment of the intestine.

Stress hormones therefore suppress digestion by shifting the system away from its coordinated sequence and reducing its capacity to process incoming food. The effects are expressed through changes in acid production, enzyme release, bile flow, motility, and blood flow. When this state persists, the digestive system operates under constrained conditions, and the consequences extend into every downstream process that depends on proper digestion.

Chapter 21

Neurological and Systemic Symptoms

Neurological and systemic symptoms arise when the digestive sequence fails to deliver a stable supply of substrates and instead produces a variable internal environment that extends beyond the intestine. The brain and peripheral systems depend on consistent inputs of glucose, amino acids, fatty acids, and micronutrients, delivered in a pattern that matches metabolic demand. When digestion is aligned, these inputs remain steady and predictable. When it is not, fluctuations in substrate availability, combined with changes in microbial output and immune signaling, propagate into the systemic circulation and alter how the body functions at multiple levels.

The first layer of this effect is substrate instability. Incomplete digestion reduces the availability of usable nutrients, while irregular absorption creates uneven timing of delivery. The brain relies on a continuous supply of substrates to maintain signaling and energy production. When this supply becomes inconsistent, neuronal activity reflects that variability. Periods of adequate substrate availability are followed by periods of relative deficit, creating fluctuations in cognitive function, focus, and overall neurological performance. The system compensates, but the compensation introduces variability rather than restoring stability.

Lipid-derived substrates play a central role in stabilizing neurological function because they provide sustained energy and contribute to membrane structure within neural tissue. When fat digestion and transport are aligned, fatty acids are delivered gradually, supporting continuous energy production and maintaining membrane composition.

When lipid processing is impaired, this sustained supply is reduced, and the system becomes more dependent on rapidly fluctuating carbohydrate-derived substrates. This increases variability in neuronal energy availability and affects signaling consistency.

Microbial activity contributes an additional layer of influence by generating compounds that enter circulation when fermentation increases. These byproducts reflect the substrates that reach the distal intestine and the metabolic activity of the microbial population. When digestion is incomplete, increased fermentation produces a wider range of compounds that interact with the systemic environment. These compounds alter signaling patterns and contribute to changes in how the nervous system responds to internal conditions.

Immune signaling links the intestinal environment to systemic responses. Increased exposure to incomplete substrates and microbial byproducts elevates signaling at the epithelial surface, and this signaling extends beyond the gut through circulating mediators. The result is a change in how the body regulates its internal state, affecting energy use, perception, and overall physiological behavior. This connection reflects the integration of digestive, immune, and neurological systems.

Hormonal responses further shape these outcomes by reacting to the variability in substrate delivery. Fluctuations in nutrient availability alter signals that regulate energy distribution, storage, and use. These changes influence how substrates are directed toward the brain and other tissues, affecting both immediate function and longer-term stability.

Neurological and systemic symptoms therefore represent the outward expression of an internal sequence that has lost consistency. They arise from fluctuations in substrate availability, changes in microbial output, and increased immune signaling, all of which originate from disrupted digestion. When the digestive sequence is restored and substrate delivery becomes stable, these downstream effects are reduced as the system returns to a more predictable internal environment.

Brain Fog, Fatigue, Inflammation

Brain fog, fatigue, and inflammation emerge from the same underlying condition, which is an unstable internal environment created by disrupted digestion and inconsistent substrate delivery. These are not isolated symptoms with separate causes. They reflect how the brain and peripheral systems respond when energy supply, molecular signaling, and immune activity are no longer aligned with the body's structural requirements. The digestive system sets the conditions, and the nervous system expresses the outcome.

Brain fog begins with variability in substrate availability. Neurons require a continuous supply of energy substrates to maintain signaling. When digestion is incomplete or absorption is irregular, the delivery of these substrates becomes uneven. Periods of adequate supply are followed by periods where availability drops, forcing the brain to adjust its activity. These shifts alter how neurons fire, how networks coordinate, and how information is processed. The result is a reduction in clarity, slower processing speed, and a sense that cognitive output no longer matches demand.

Fatigue develops from the same instability but reflects the system at a broader level. When substrates are not delivered consistently, cells across the body must adjust their energy production to match what is available. Mitochondria shift between fuels, alter pathway activity, and operate under changing conditions. This constant adjustment reduces efficiency and increases variability in energy output. The body compensates by reducing activity, conserving resources, and limiting output where possible. Fatigue is the expression of this constraint, not simply a lack of energy but an inability to sustain stable production.

Inflammation links these symptoms by responding to the internal conditions created by incomplete digestion. Larger food fragments and microbial byproducts increase signaling at the intestinal interface, and this signaling extends into circulation. The immune system reacts to the presence of these materials by altering its activity, producing a state where signaling is elevated and persistent. This state changes how tissues function, how energy is used, and how the nervous system interprets internal signals.

Lipid processing plays a stabilizing role across all three conditions. When fats are properly emulsified, absorbed, and transported, they provide a sustained source of energy and contribute to the structural integrity of cellular membranes. This supports consistent energy production and stable signaling. When lipid digestion is impaired, this stabilizing influence is reduced, and the system becomes more dependent on rapidly fluctuating substrates. The variability increases, and the symptoms become more pronounced.

The interaction between these processes creates a feedback pattern. Inconsistent substrate delivery alters energy production, changes in energy production affect cellular function, and immune signaling modifies the internal environment further. Each layer influences the others, reinforcing the instability that produced the initial symptoms.

Brain fog, fatigue, and inflammation therefore represent different expressions of the same underlying disruption. They arise when digestion fails to provide a stable and complete supply of substrates, when microbial activity shifts due to incomplete processing, and when immune signaling responds to the resulting environment. Restoring the digestive sequence changes the inputs to the system, and as those inputs stabilize, the downstream effects begin to resolve in parallel.

Gut–Brain Signaling Breakdown

Gut–brain signaling depends on a continuous exchange of information that reflects the state of digestion, the availability of substrates, and the condition of the intestinal environment. This exchange is carried through neural pathways, circulating metabolites, and immune signals that originate at the epithelial surface. When digestion is aligned, these signals are proportional to real conditions and allow the brain to coordinate appetite, energy use, and behavioral output with what is actually available. When digestion is disrupted, the signals no longer represent a stable internal state. The brain receives inconsistent inputs and responds to a system that is changing from moment to moment.

The breakdown begins with variability in luminal processing. Incomplete digestion increases the presence of larger food fragments and shifts microbial activity toward fermentation. This alters the profile of compounds generated within the intestine. These compounds enter circulation or interact with neural pathways embedded in the gut wall, changing the signals that are sent to the brain. The pattern becomes irregular because it reflects inconsistent processing rather than a controlled sequence.

Neural signaling through the gut is highly sensitive to mechanical and chemical conditions. Distension, pressure, and the composition of luminal contents all influence how signals are generated. When motility is coordinated and substrates are properly processed, these inputs remain within a narrow range. When digestion is incomplete, gas production increases, pressure fluctuates, and the physical state of the intestine becomes more variable. Neural signals track these changes, transmitting a pattern that reflects instability rather than balance.

Circulating signals add another layer to this breakdown. Substrates that are absorbed enter the bloodstream and influence how the brain interprets internal conditions. When absorption is consistent, these signals provide a reliable representation of nutrient availability. When absorption is irregular, the signals fluctuate, and the brain must respond to changing conditions. This affects how energy is allocated and how behavior is regulated.

Immune signaling integrates with both neural and circulating pathways. Increased exposure to incomplete substrates and microbial byproducts elevates activity at the intestinal interface. This activity generates signals that extend beyond the gut, altering the overall signaling environment. The brain interprets these signals as part of the body's internal state, adjusting its output accordingly.

Lipid transport influences gut–brain signaling by shaping the timing and persistence of substrate delivery. When lipid digestion and transport are aligned, fatty acids enter circulation in a sustained pattern that supports stable signaling. When this process is impaired, the system becomes dominated by more rapidly fluctuating inputs, increasing variability in how signals are generated and interpreted.

Gut–brain signaling breakdown therefore reflects a loss of alignment between digestion and communication. Signals are still produced, but they no longer correspond to a stable or predictable internal state. The brain responds to this variability, adjusting behavior and physiological output to match inputs that are inconsistent. Restoring the digestive sequence reestablishes the conditions under which signals accurately represent internal reality, allowing coordination between the gut and brain to stabilize.

PART X

RESTORING DIGESTIVE ORDER

Chapter 22

Restoring the Digestive State

Restoring the digestive state requires reestablishing the conditions under which the system can operate in sequence. Digestion does not begin with food composition. It begins with permission. The nervous system determines whether the body allocates resources toward processing incoming material or diverts those resources elsewhere. When this state is constrained, acid production declines, enzyme release weakens, bile flow becomes inconsistent, and motility loses coordination. The goal is not to force output at isolated points but to restore the upstream conditions that allow the entire sequence to activate as a single system.

The first layer of restoration occurs at the level of neural input. Sensory engagement with food initiates the cephalic phase, which prepares the stomach, pancreas, and biliary system before swallowing occurs. This phase is mechanical and predictable. When food is seen, smelled, and tasted under conditions of low stress, signals are sent that increase secretory output and coordinate downstream activity. When this phase is absent or reduced, the system begins in a weakened state. Restoring it means allowing sufficient time and attention for these signals to form before food enters the stomach.

Pacing reshapes how these signals are maintained. Rapid intake compresses the digestive sequence, forcing multiple phases to overlap without proper transition. The stomach receives material before it is fully prepared, and downstream organs respond to incomplete signals. Slowing the rate of intake extends the time over which signals are generated and sustained. This allows acid production to reach effective levels, enzymes to be released in proportion to substrate load, and bile flow to align with lipid arrival. The sequence regains structure because each step has the time required to activate and complete its role.

Mechanical processing in the mouth contributes directly to restoration by reducing particle size and increasing surface area. This change is not only physical. It alters how the stomach perceives incoming material and how quickly it can act on it. Smaller, well-processed particles allow acid to interact more uniformly, supporting protein unfolding and preparing substrates for enzymatic cleavage. This reduces the burden on downstream processes and improves the efficiency of the entire sequence.

Gastric conditions must be allowed to develop fully. Acid production is not instantaneous. It increases in response to incoming signals and substrate presence. When intake is rushed or when prior phases are weak, acid levels may not reach the threshold required to properly modify food structure. Allowing sufficient time between intake and progression to the next phase ensures that proteins are unfolded and that the material entering the small intestine is in a state that can be further processed.

Coordination between the stomach and small intestine defines whether the sequence continues or breaks down. The release of gastric contents must match the capacity of the intestine to process them. When this coordination is restored, substrates enter in controlled amounts that can be matched by enzyme release and bile flow. When it is not, the intestine receives material that exceeds its processing capacity, leading to incomplete digestion and downstream effects. Restoration focuses on reestablishing this balance so that delivery and processing remain aligned.

Lipid digestion plays a central role in stabilizing the restored state because it provides a sustained input that extends beyond the rapid phases of carbohydrate processing. When fats are properly emulsified and absorbed, they create a prolonged delivery of substrates that supports steady energy production and consistent signaling. This stabilizes the system and reduces variability in downstream responses. Ensuring that bile flow and emulsification occur in coordination with lipid intake is therefore a key part of restoring overall function.

Restoring the digestive state is not achieved by targeting individual symptoms or isolated steps. It requires rebuilding the sequence from the beginning so that each phase prepares the next. Neural input initiates the process, mechanical and chemical preparation in the stomach establishes substrate structure, coordinated release aligns with intestinal capacity, and transport systems deliver nutrients in a controlled pattern. When these elements are reconnected, the system returns to a state where digestion proceeds as an integrated function rather than a series of disconnected events.

Nervous System Regulation

Nervous system regulation defines whether digestion is allowed to operate as a coordinated sequence or remains constrained at every level. The digestive system does not function independently. It is governed by neural inputs that determine blood flow, secretion, motility, and timing before any chemical processing begins. When these inputs are aligned, the system transitions into a state where resources are directed toward digestion. When they are not, output is reduced regardless of food composition or nutrient density. Regulation at this level sets the ceiling for everything that follows.

The transition into a digestive state begins with parasympathetic activation, which increases secretory output and organizes motility into patterns that support mixing and controlled progression. Gastric acid production rises, pancreatic enzymes are released in proportion to incoming substrates, and bile flow aligns with lipid presence. These responses are coordinated through neural signaling that integrates sensory input with internal conditions. When this activation is incomplete, each of these outputs is reduced. The stomach produces less acid, the pancreas releases fewer enzymes, and bile delivery becomes inconsistent. The sequence weakens before it has fully begun.

Sympathetic activation produces the opposite effect by reallocating resources away from digestion. Blood flow to the gastrointestinal tract decreases, limiting both secretion and absorption. Motility patterns shift, often becoming irregular or accelerated in ways that reduce contact time between substrates and enzymes. This changes how material is processed and where it accumulates within the system. The reduction in perfusion also affects the epithelial surface, decreasing the efficiency of transport systems that move nutrients into circulation. These changes occur together, creating a state where the digestive system operates under constraint.

Regulation is not binary. It exists along a range, and the digestive system responds proportionally to the degree of activation. Partial activation produces partial output. This creates a condition where digestion may appear functional but operates below capacity. Substrates are processed incompletely, signals are weakened, and downstream effects begin to accumulate. The system adapts to this reduced state, but the adaptation reflects limitation rather than restoration.

Neural regulation also determines how signals propagate through the sequence. Early-phase signaling from sensory input influences gastric activity, which in turn shapes pancreatic and biliary responses. When the initial signals are weak, the downstream responses are proportionally reduced. This propagation effect means that small changes in neural input at the beginning of the sequence can produce larger changes in output later on. Restoring regulation at the top of the sequence therefore has amplified effects throughout the system.

Lipid digestion depends heavily on this regulation because bile release and coordinated motility are required to process fats effectively. When neural input supports proper timing and flow, lipids are emulsified and absorbed in a pattern that stabilizes energy delivery and signaling. When regulation is impaired, this coordination breaks down, reducing lipid processing and removing a stabilizing influence on the system.

Nervous system regulation therefore acts as the primary control layer for digestion. It determines whether the system operates with full capacity, partial output, or suppression. Restoring this regulation aligns blood flow, secretion, motility, and timing, allowing the digestive sequence to function as an integrated process. When this control layer is stable, the downstream processes it governs regain their structure and efficiency.

Re-establishing Parasympathetic Dominance

Re-establishing parasympathetic dominance means restoring the internal conditions under which digestion is permitted to run as a full sequence rather than a constrained process. The parasympathetic state is not an abstract relaxation response. It is a specific physiological configuration where blood flow is directed toward the gastrointestinal tract, secretory activity increases, and motility organizes into patterns that support mixing, breakdown, and controlled progression. When this state is absent or only partially activated, digestion proceeds with reduced output at every level. The goal is to shift the system back into a state where these processes can occur without restriction.

The transition begins with sensory engagement and pacing. The cephalic phase depends on visual, olfactory, and gustatory input to initiate digestive signaling before food enters the stomach. When meals are approached without interruption and with sufficient attention, these signals activate neural pathways that increase gastric acid production and prepare downstream organs. This is a mechanical process. The presence of food cues under low-stress conditions generates predictable changes in output. When this phase is compressed or bypassed, the system starts in a weakened state and must attempt to catch up after food has already entered the stomach.

Breathing patterns directly influence this transition by altering autonomic balance. Slower, controlled breathing increases parasympathetic input and reduces competing signals that suppress digestive activity. This change affects heart rate, vascular tone, and neural signaling to the gastrointestinal tract. As parasympathetic influence increases, blood flow to digestive organs rises, supporting secretion and absorption. The effect is not isolated to one organ. It shifts the entire system toward a configuration that favors processing incoming material.

Posture and physical positioning contribute to how this state is maintained. An upright and stable position supports coordinated motility and reduces mechanical constraints on the stomach and intestines. When the body is compressed or moving rapidly, signals that support digestion are reduced, and motility patterns become less organized. Maintaining a stable position during intake allows neural signaling to remain consistent and supports the mechanical aspects of digestion.

Consistency reinforces this state over time. The nervous system adapts to repeated patterns of input. When meals are consistently approached under conditions that favor parasympathetic activation, the system begins to anticipate and prepare for digestion more effectively. Secretory responses become more proportional, motility patterns stabilize, and coordination between organs improves. This adaptation reflects repeated exposure to conditions that allow the sequence to run as designed.

Lipid digestion highlights the importance of sustained parasympathetic activity because bile release and emulsification depend on coordinated signaling over time. When this state is maintained, fats are processed efficiently and provide a prolonged supply of substrates that support stable energy production. When it is not, bile flow becomes inconsistent, and lipid processing is reduced, removing a key stabilizing input to the system.

Re-establishing parasympathetic dominance therefore restores the foundational state required for digestion to operate as a coordinated system. It aligns neural input with the structural and functional demands of the digestive sequence, allowing each phase to activate in order and at sufficient capacity. When this state is consistent, the system regains its ability to process food effectively, and the downstream effects that depend on proper digestion begin to stabilize.

Chapter 23

Rebuilding Sequence

Rebuilding the digestive sequence requires restoring the order, timing, and dependency relationships that define how digestion operates as a system. Each phase prepares the next. When that order is disrupted, downstream processes are forced to operate on substrates that do not match their requirements, and compensation begins to replace coordination. The objective is not to correct isolated failures but to reestablish the chain of preparation so that each step receives the correct input at the correct time. Sequence is the mechanism that converts intake into usable output. Without it, digestion becomes fragmented and inefficient.

The starting point is the reestablishment of early-phase signaling. Sensory input initiates the cascade that drives gastric and pancreatic output, and this input must be present and sustained long enough to generate a full response. When this phase is restored, the stomach enters a state where acid production rises in proportion to the incoming load, creating the conditions required for structural modification of proteins. This step determines whether downstream enzymes will be able to act efficiently. If proteins remain folded and resistant, the rest of the sequence inherits that limitation.

Gastric processing defines the structural state of all incoming material. Acid exposure unfolds proteins, alters physical properties of the food matrix, and sets the rate at which contents are released into the small intestine. Rebuilding sequence at this level means allowing gastric conditions to develop fully before progression occurs. When this is achieved, the material entering the intestine is already partially processed and aligned with the requirements of enzymatic breakdown. When it is not, the intestine receives material that is structurally incomplete, and processing capacity is exceeded.

The transition between the stomach and small intestine must be re-synchronized so that delivery matches processing capacity. Gastric emptying is not a passive event. It is regulated based on the condition of the contents and the readiness of the intestine to receive them. Rebuilding this transition means restoring the feedback signals that control release. When these signals are functioning, substrates enter the intestine in controlled amounts that can be matched by enzyme secretion and bile flow. This prevents overload and maintains alignment between delivery and processing.

Pancreatic enzyme release and bile flow operate as a coupled system within the intestine. Enzymes reduce macromolecules into smaller components, while bile organizes lipids into structures that can be accessed and absorbed. Rebuilding sequence here requires that both systems activate in proportion to the incoming substrate load. When they are synchronized, breakdown proceeds efficiently and absorption can occur without accumulation of partially processed material. When they are not, incomplete substrates move forward, and downstream regions compensate through microbial metabolism.

Absorption and transport complete the sequence by moving processed substrates into circulation and distributing them to tissues. This step depends on the prior phases having produced the correct molecular forms. Rebuilding sequence ensures that transport systems receive substrates they can handle, allowing for efficient uptake and delivery. Lipid transport, in particular, provides a sustained flow of substrates that stabilizes energy availability and supports consistent signaling across systems.

The rebuilding process also requires removing patterns that disrupt sequence. Rapid intake, inconsistent pacing, and irregular timing compress phases that should remain distinct. This compression forces multiple steps to occur simultaneously without proper preparation, weakening the entire chain. Restoring sequence separates these phases again, allowing each to complete its function before the next begins.

Rebuilding sequence therefore reestablishes digestion as an ordered system where structure leads to function and function leads to output. Early signaling prepares the system, gastric processing modifies substrate structure, controlled release aligns with intestinal capacity, enzymatic and biliary activity complete breakdown, and transport delivers nutrients in a stable pattern. When these steps are restored in order, digestion returns to a state where each phase supports the next, and the system operates as a coordinated whole rather than a series of compensations.

Acid → Bile → Enzymes → Motility

This sequence defines the operational order of digestion, where each phase sets the conditions required for the next to function correctly. It is not a list of independent components. It is a dependency chain. When the order is preserved, digestion proceeds with coordination and efficiency. When it is disrupted, downstream processes receive substrates that do not match their requirements, and the system shifts into compensation rather than alignment.

Gastric acid establishes the structural state of incoming food. Proteins are unfolded, connective structures are loosened, and the physical matrix of the meal is altered in a way that increases access for downstream enzymes. This step determines whether enzymatic cleavage can occur efficiently. When acid exposure is sufficient, substrates are reduced into forms that can be processed further. When it is not, larger and more resistant structures persist, limiting the ability of enzymes to act and setting a constraint that carries forward through the entire sequence.

Bile follows as the structural organizer of lipids. Once gastric processing has reduced and dispersed the meal, bile interacts with lipid components to break them into smaller, uniformly distributed structures. This increases surface area and allows enzymes to access and act on fats effectively. Without this step, lipids remain in larger aggregates that resist enzymatic action. The presence and timing of bile therefore determine whether fat processing proceeds efficiently or becomes a limiting factor in the sequence.

Enzymes act on substrates that have already been structurally prepared by acid and bile. Proteases, lipases, and other enzymes require access to specific molecular configurations. When upstream processing has occurred, enzymes can rapidly reduce macromolecules into absorbable units. When it has not, their activity is restricted, and breakdown remains incomplete. Enzymes do not compensate for poor preparation. They operate within the constraints defined by earlier phases.

Motility governs how substrates move through this sequence and whether each phase has sufficient time to act. Coordinated motility patterns mix contents, distribute enzymes and bile, and regulate the rate at which material progresses through the system. When motility is aligned, substrates remain in contact with the components required for processing, and each phase completes its function before progression occurs. When motility is disrupted, material may move too quickly, reducing contact time, or too slowly, increasing exposure to partially processed substrates and altering the internal environment.

The sequence functions as a continuous flow where structure determines access, access determines breakdown, and breakdown determines absorption. Acid prepares, bile organizes, enzymes cleave, and motility coordinates. Each step depends on the one before it, and failure at any point alters the conditions for everything that follows.

Rebuilding this sequence restores digestion as an ordered process rather than a fragmented one. When acid production is sufficient, bile flow is coordinated, enzymatic activity matches substrate load, and motility maintains proper timing, the system converts intake into usable output with consistency. When any part of this chain is weakened, the effects propagate forward, reducing efficiency and increasing variability in downstream outcomes.

Why Order Matters More Than Inputs

Order determines whether inputs can be used at all. The digestive system is not designed to handle raw inputs in any form at any time. It is designed to transform them through a sequence where each step changes the structure of the material and prepares it for the next operation. When that order is preserved, even variable inputs can be processed effectively because each phase receives substrates that match its requirements. When the order is disrupted, even high-quality inputs fail to be utilized because they arrive in forms that the system cannot handle.

The constraint is structural. Gastric acid must act before enzymes can access proteins, bile must organize lipids before they can be broken down and absorbed, and transport systems can only move molecules that fall within specific size and polarity ranges. These are not preferences. They are physical requirements. If a step is skipped or weakened, the substrate remains outside the range that downstream processes can act on. No increase in input quality changes this. The system cannot bypass structural preparation.

Timing reinforces this dependency. Each phase requires a specific window to act on incoming material. When intake is rushed or when transitions between phases are compressed, multiple processes overlap without completion. The stomach releases material that has not been fully processed, the intestine receives more than it can handle at once, and enzymes operate on substrates that are not ready. This creates a condition where inputs are present but not usable, and a portion of those inputs moves through the system without being captured.

Transport systems further enforce the importance of order. Absorption is selective. Molecules must be reduced to defined forms before they can cross the intestinal membrane. Larger fragments, poorly organized lipids, and partially processed carbohydrates remain in the lumen regardless of their origin or quality. The presence of these materials does not contribute to the internal substrate pool. They are effectively excluded from the system.

When order is preserved, the same inputs produce a different outcome because they are transformed in sequence. Proteins are unfolded and cleaved into amino acids, lipids are emulsified and reduced into absorbable units, and carbohydrates are processed into simple sugars. These forms can be transported, distributed, and used by cells. The system extracts value because each phase prepares the next, and the entire chain operates without interruption.

When order is disrupted, the system shifts into compensation. Downstream regions attempt to process material that should have been handled earlier, microbial activity increases to metabolize what remains, and immune signaling responds to the presence of incomplete substrates. These responses do not restore the original sequence. They reflect an attempt to manage a condition where inputs are present but improperly prepared.

Order therefore defines whether inputs become usable outputs. It sets the conditions under which digestion converts food into substrates that can be absorbed and utilized. Changing inputs without restoring order leaves the underlying constraint in place. Restoring order changes how those inputs are processed, allowing the system to operate according to its design and extract value from what is consumed.

Chapter 24

Increasing Digestive Capacity

Increasing digestive capacity means expanding how much the system can process, transform, and absorb without breakdown or compensation. Capacity is not fixed. It is built from the alignment of neural input, secretory output, structural preparation, and coordinated timing. When these layers are functioning together, the system can handle larger and more complex inputs because each phase receives substrates that match its requirements. When they are not aligned, capacity contracts. The system may still process food, but only within a narrower range, and excess input moves forward without being fully utilized.

The first determinant of capacity is neural regulation. The level of parasympathetic activation sets the upper limit for secretion and coordination. When neural input supports digestion, gastric acid production increases, pancreatic enzymes are released in proportion to intake, and bile flow aligns with lipid presence. Blood flow to the gastrointestinal tract rises, supporting both secretion and absorption. This creates the conditions under which capacity can expand. When neural input is constrained, these outputs are reduced, and the system operates below its potential regardless of how much food is consumed.

Structural preparation defines how efficiently substrates can be processed. Gastric acid unfolds proteins and alters the physical state of the meal, increasing access for enzymes. Bile organizes lipids into dispersed structures that can be acted on and absorbed. When these preparatory steps are complete, downstream processes operate with less resistance and greater efficiency. This effectively increases capacity because the same enzymatic and transport systems can process a larger amount of substrate when it is properly prepared.

Enzymatic activity determines the rate at which macromolecules are reduced into absorbable forms. When enzyme release matches substrate load, breakdown proceeds continuously, and accumulation of partially processed material is minimized. When release is insufficient or poorly timed, substrates exceed the system's ability to process them, and capacity appears limited. Increasing capacity at this level requires aligning enzyme output with the volume and type of incoming material, ensuring that breakdown keeps pace with delivery.

Motility and timing govern how long substrates remain within each phase of digestion and how effectively they are mixed with digestive components. Coordinated motility patterns ensure that substrates remain in contact with acid, enzymes, and bile long enough for processing to occur. When timing is aligned, each phase completes its function before progression. When it is not, material may move too quickly, reducing processing time, or too slowly, increasing exposure to incomplete substrates and altering the internal environment. Capacity expands when timing allows each phase to operate fully.

Lipid digestion plays a stabilizing role in capacity because it provides a sustained flow of substrates that supports continuous energy production and consistent signaling. When fats are properly emulsified and absorbed, they extend the delivery of energy beyond the rapid phases of carbohydrate processing. This reduces variability in substrate availability and allows the system to operate at a higher level without fluctuation. When lipid processing is impaired, this stabilizing input is reduced, and capacity becomes more dependent on rapidly changing conditions.

Absorption and transport complete the expansion of capacity by determining how efficiently processed substrates are moved into circulation. When transport systems receive substrates in the correct form and at a rate they can handle, uptake proceeds continuously. When substrates arrive in forms that do not match transport requirements or in amounts that exceed capacity, absorption becomes a limiting factor. Improving capacity at this stage depends on the alignment of upstream processes that deliver substrates in a usable form.

Increasing digestive capacity therefore requires restoring and strengthening the sequence that governs digestion. Neural activation sets the conditions, structural preparation reduces resistance, enzymatic activity completes breakdown, motility maintains timing, and transport delivers substrates into the system. When these elements are aligned, the system expands its ability to process input and convert it into usable output. Capacity is not increased by forcing more input into the system but by improving how that input is prepared, processed, and absorbed.

Gradual System Reloading

Gradual system reloading restores digestive capacity by increasing input in a way that matches the system's current processing ability while allowing each phase of the sequence to strengthen. After a period of constrained digestion, the system adapts to lower output. Acid production, enzyme release, bile flow, and motility operate at reduced levels because demand has been low or inconsistent. Introducing a large substrate load into this state overwhelms the sequence immediately. Substrates exceed processing capacity, incomplete material accumulates, and downstream effects reappear. Reloading avoids this by scaling input to the system's present capacity and expanding that capacity over time.

The process begins with controlling substrate load per exposure. Smaller, well-defined inputs allow gastric acid to reach effective levels relative to the amount of protein present, enabling full structural modification before progression. This creates substrates that downstream enzymes can access without resistance. As this pattern repeats, acid production adapts upward because the system is repeatedly asked to meet a slightly higher but still manageable demand. The increase is incremental, and each step reinforces the next.

Lipid introduction follows the same principle but with additional dependence on bile coordination. Moderate amounts of fat stimulate bile release and establish the timing relationship between gastric emptying and intestinal processing. When lipid input matches the system's ability to emulsify and absorb, fats are processed efficiently and provide a sustained substrate flow that stabilizes energy delivery. Increasing lipid load gradually allows bile production and release patterns to adapt without creating accumulation of poorly processed fats in the intestine.

Enzymatic capacity expands in response to repeated exposure to substrates that have been properly prepared. When proteins are unfolded and lipids are emulsified, enzymes operate efficiently and complete breakdown within the available time window. Repeated successful processing reinforces enzyme release patterns and maintains alignment between substrate load and catalytic activity. Increasing input too quickly disrupts this alignment, forcing enzymes to operate on substrates that exceed their capacity or are not structurally prepared.

Motility adapts alongside these changes by maintaining coordinated movement that matches the rate of processing. Smaller, controlled inputs allow mixing and progression to remain synchronized with enzymatic activity. As input increases gradually, motility patterns adjust to handle larger volumes without losing coordination. This preserves contact time between substrates and digestive components, preventing the premature movement of partially processed material.

Transport systems complete the reloading process by absorbing substrates that have been fully reduced. When inputs are scaled appropriately, transport occurs continuously without saturation. This reinforces the entire sequence because successful absorption reduces the accumulation of material within the lumen and supports stable delivery of nutrients into circulation. As capacity increases upstream, transport adapts to handle the increased flow.

Gradual system reloading therefore rebuilds digestive capacity by aligning input with current function and expanding that function through repeated, successful processing. Each phase is reinforced in sequence. Acid prepares, bile organizes, enzymes complete breakdown, motility maintains timing, and transport delivers substrates into the system. Increasing input only after these steps are operating effectively allows capacity to grow without triggering the same failures that reduced it.

Expanding Food Tolerance

Food tolerance expands when the digestive system regains the ability to fully process a wider range of substrates and deliver them in forms the body can use without triggering compensation. Tolerance is not a property of the food itself. It is a function of capacity. When digestion is aligned, proteins are reduced to amino acids, carbohydrates are converted to simple sugars, and lipids are emulsified and absorbed in a controlled pattern. These forms pass through the intestinal barrier without generating excess immune signaling. When digestion is incomplete, larger fragments and poorly processed substrates remain in the lumen, increasing the likelihood that the system reacts to their presence. Expanding tolerance therefore requires improving how inputs are processed, not simply changing which inputs are consumed.

The first step is restoring structural preparation so that substrates entering the intestine match the requirements of enzymes and transport systems. Adequate gastric acid unfolds proteins and reduces the physical resistance of the meal. Coordinated bile release organizes lipids into dispersed structures that can be accessed and absorbed. When these steps are consistent, downstream processes operate with less friction, and a greater proportion of the meal is converted into usable forms. This reduces the amount of material that reaches distal regions in a partially processed state.

Timing and pacing determine whether this preparation is maintained as input increases. Smaller, controlled exposures allow the system to process substrates completely before introducing additional load. As capacity improves, the range and quantity of inputs can expand without exceeding processing ability. Each successful exposure reinforces the sequence, allowing the system to handle more complex or previously problematic foods. Increasing input too quickly disrupts this progression, reintroducing incomplete processing and limiting tolerance.

Lipid digestion contributes to tolerance by stabilizing the internal environment of the intestine. Properly emulsified and absorbed fats provide a sustained source of substrates and influence how other nutrients are processed. This stabilizing effect reduces variability in substrate delivery and supports consistent signaling across the system. When lipid processing is impaired, this stability is reduced, and tolerance becomes more sensitive to changes in input.

Microbial activity reflects the state of digestion and influences tolerance indirectly. When substrates are fully processed and absorbed, less material reaches distal regions for fermentation. When digestion is incomplete, increased fermentation alters the internal environment and contributes to variability in how the system responds to food. Improving upstream processing reduces this substrate load and shifts microbial activity toward a pattern that supports stability rather than variability.

Immune signaling decreases as processing improves because fewer incomplete fragments reach the intestinal interface. The barrier is exposed to substrates that match transport requirements rather than larger or irregular structures. This reduces the signals that drive reactivity and allows tolerance to expand. The change is not achieved by suppressing the immune response but by reducing the conditions that provoke it.

Expanding food tolerance therefore follows from restoring the digestive sequence and increasing capacity in a controlled manner. Structural preparation, coordinated timing, enzymatic breakdown, and efficient transport convert a broader range of inputs into usable outputs. As this process stabilizes, the system handles more foods without triggering downstream effects, and tolerance reflects the improved function of the digestive system rather than the restriction of inputs.

Chapter 25

Supplements for Support

Supplementation functions as a support layer that interacts with the digestive sequence rather than replacing it. Each compound or category of support targets a specific phase, and its effectiveness depends on whether that phase is active and able to respond. When the sequence is aligned, supplements can increase output, improve coordination, and reduce the gap between current capacity and demand. When the sequence is suppressed, the same inputs produce limited effects because the system they act on is not operating at full function. The role of supplementation is therefore conditional. It amplifies an existing process or stabilizes a weak point within the sequence, but it does not create a new pathway.

The most effective support aligns with the order of digestion, beginning with neural activation and early-phase signaling. Compounds that stimulate sensory pathways, such as bitter agonists, increase vagal input and elevate gastric acid, enzyme release, and bile flow. This strengthens the initial transition into a digestive state and improves the quality of the inputs entering downstream phases. When this step is reinforced, the rest of the sequence operates on substrates that are closer to the required structural form, reducing the burden on later processes.

Gastric support focuses on restoring the conditions required for protein transformation and overall meal processing. When acid production is insufficient relative to the incoming load, structural preparation remains incomplete. Targeted support at this level increases the capacity of the stomach to modify substrates before they progress. This changes how enzymes interact with proteins and how the small intestine receives and processes incoming material. The effect is amplified when upstream signaling is already active, because acid production responds to both neural input and substrate presence.

Pancreatic enzyme support provides direct catalytic activity that assists in reducing macromolecules into absorbable units. This is most effective when substrates have already been structurally prepared by gastric acid and dispersed by bile. Under those conditions, supplemental enzymes integrate into the existing breakdown process and increase the rate and completeness of cleavage. When structural preparation is incomplete, their activity is constrained, and the effect is reduced. Enzyme support therefore depends on the integrity of the phases that precede it.

Bile support targets the organization and absorption of lipids within the small intestine. When endogenous bile release is insufficient or poorly timed, supplemental bile improves emulsification and increases the formation of absorbable lipid structures. This enhances the delivery of fatty acids and fat-soluble nutrients and stabilizes energy availability. The impact extends beyond fat digestion because lipid processing influences the overall environment of the intestine and the timing of substrate delivery into circulation.

Absorptive and transport support operates at the final stage of the sequence, where processed substrates are moved into the body. Compounds that influence membrane function, transport efficiency, or luminal conditions can improve the rate at which nutrients are captured. This support is effective only when upstream processing has produced substrates in the correct form. When larger or improperly processed molecules remain, transport systems cannot compensate, and the benefit is limited.

The interaction between these layers reflects the dependency chain of digestion. Support applied in sequence reinforces each phase in order, allowing the system to operate with greater efficiency and stability. When applied out of sequence, support becomes fragmented and less effective because the underlying structure required for full digestion is not present.

Supplementation therefore acts as a targeted input into a larger system, enhancing capacity where the system is already capable of responding. Its role is to support alignment, improve efficiency, and reduce the gap between current function and optimal output. When the digestive sequence is restored and supplements are used in accordance with that sequence, they integrate into the system and amplify its performance rather than attempting to replace it.

Digestive Bitters

Digestive bitters act at the very beginning of the digestive sequence by triggering sensory pathways that initiate downstream activity before food is processed. Their primary effect is neural. Bitter compounds activate receptors in the mouth and upper gastrointestinal tract, sending signals through vagal pathways that increase gastric acid production, pancreatic enzyme release, and bile flow. This occurs prior to swallowing and sets the initial conditions under which the rest of digestion will operate. When this signal is strong, the system enters the meal in an active state rather than attempting to generate output after food has already arrived.

The effect of bitters is proportional to the system's ability to respond. When parasympathetic input is present and the digestive organs are capable of increasing output, bitters sharpen and accelerate the onset of secretion. Gastric acid rises more quickly relative to the incoming protein load, improving structural preparation. Pancreatic output aligns more closely with substrate arrival, and bile release becomes more coordinated with lipid intake. This alignment reduces the lag between intake and processing, allowing each phase to begin with sufficient capacity already in place.

Bitters influence timing as much as magnitude. By strengthening early-phase signaling, they extend the window during which digestive processes are active and coordinated. This affects how long acid remains elevated, how enzymes are released over the course of a meal, and how bile flow is sustained. The result is a more continuous and stable processing environment rather than a delayed or compressed response. When early signaling is weak, downstream phases attempt to compensate after the fact, often with reduced efficiency.

The structural impact of this signaling becomes apparent in how substrates are handled. Proteins entering a stomach that has already increased acid output are unfolded more completely and more rapidly. This creates substrates that enzymes can access without resistance. Lipids entering an intestine that has already initiated bile flow are emulsified more effectively, improving enzyme contact and absorption. Bitters do not directly break down food. They prepare the system so that breakdown can occur efficiently.

The effectiveness of bitters is limited when the system is suppressed. If neural input is constrained or if secretory capacity is reduced, the signal generated by bitter receptors does not translate into a full downstream response. In this state, bitters may produce only a partial increase in output, and the sequence remains incomplete. Their role is to amplify an existing pathway, not to replace it.

Repeated use under conditions that allow a full response can reinforce the digestive sequence over time. The nervous system adapts to consistent patterns of activation, and the relationship between sensory input and digestive output becomes more reliable. This improves the predictability of acid production, enzyme release, and bile flow with each exposure.

Digestive bitters therefore function as a signal that initiates and strengthens the digestive sequence at its earliest point. They increase the speed and coordination of the transition into an active digestive state, allowing subsequent phases to operate with greater efficiency. Their effect depends on the system's capacity to respond, and when that capacity is present, they improve how the entire sequence begins and unfolds.

Ox Bile, TUDCA

Ox bile and TUDCA operate within the lipid phase of digestion, but they influence different layers of the system. Ox bile functions directly in the intestinal lumen as a structural agent that organizes fats into forms that can be processed and absorbed. TUDCA functions at the level of bile composition and flow, influencing how bile is produced, transported, and maintained within the system. Both affect lipid handling, but their roles are not interchangeable. One acts on the substrate in the intestine, while the other acts on the system that generates and moves bile.

Ox bile supplements introduce bile acids into the small intestine at the time lipids arrive. These bile acids interact with dietary fats, breaking larger lipid aggregates into smaller, dispersed structures that increase surface area. This allows pancreatic lipases to access triglycerides and reduce them into absorbable components. The effect is immediate and mechanical. When endogenous bile release is insufficient or poorly timed, ox bile compensates by providing the structural capacity required for emulsification. This improves the formation of micelles and increases the transport of fatty acids and fat-soluble nutrients across the intestinal membrane. Its effectiveness depends on coordination with gastric emptying and enzyme activity. If lipids arrive in a poorly prepared state or enzyme activity is low, the benefit is reduced because emulsification alone does not complete digestion.

TUDCA operates upstream by influencing bile flow and stability. As a taurine-conjugated bile acid, it integrates into the bile acid pool and affects how bile is synthesized, transported, and maintained. This alters the consistency of bile delivery into the intestine over time. When bile flow is irregular or constrained, TUDCA supports a more continuous and stable release, improving how lipids are processed across multiple meals rather than acting only at the moment of intake. Its effect is not limited to the lumen. It changes the internal handling of bile, influencing how the system maintains and recycles its bile acid pool.

The distinction between immediate structural support and systemic flow becomes clear when both are considered within the sequence of digestion. Ox bile acts at the point where lipids must be physically organized for enzymatic breakdown. TUDCA acts before that point by improving the system that supplies bile to the intestine. When bile production and flow are already aligned, TUDCA reinforces stability and reduces variability. When bile delivery at a given meal is insufficient, ox bile provides direct support to the emulsification process.

Lipid digestion depends on the integration of both structure and timing. Bile must be present when lipids arrive, and it must be present in sufficient quantity and composition to organize them effectively. When this coordination is achieved, fats are processed efficiently and contribute to a sustained delivery of substrates that stabilize energy production and signaling. When it is not, lipids remain in larger aggregates, limiting enzyme access and reducing absorption.

Ox bile and TUDCA therefore support lipid digestion at different points within the same system. Ox bile provides immediate structural capacity within the intestine, while TUDCA supports the upstream processes that regulate bile availability and flow. Their effectiveness depends on how well they align with the digestive sequence and with each other. When used in a system that is already coordinated, they enhance lipid processing and stabilize downstream outcomes. When the sequence is disrupted, their effects are partial because the conditions required for full lipid digestion remain incomplete.

Digestive Enzymes

Digestive enzymes function as the catalytic layer of the digestive sequence, converting structurally prepared substrates into forms that can cross the intestinal barrier. Their activity depends on what has already been done to the food. They do not initiate digestion. They complete it. When gastric acid has unfolded proteins and bile has organized lipids, enzymes can access specific bonds within these molecules and reduce them into absorbable units. When that preparation is incomplete, enzymes encounter substrates that resist cleavage, and their activity is constrained regardless of how much is present.

Proteolytic enzymes act on proteins that have been denatured by gastric acid. This unfolding exposes peptide bonds, allowing enzymes to cleave them into smaller peptides and amino acids. When acid exposure is sufficient, this process proceeds rapidly and continuously. When it is not, proteins retain structural resistance, and enzymatic breakdown slows. The result is the persistence of larger fragments that cannot be absorbed and that move downstream into regions where they alter the internal environment.

Lipolytic enzymes operate on lipids that have been dispersed by bile into smaller droplets. This dispersion increases surface area and allows enzymes to access triglycerides effectively. Without adequate emulsification, lipids remain in larger aggregates, and enzyme contact is limited. Even high levels of enzyme activity cannot compensate for poor substrate organization. The sequence must be intact for enzymes to function at full capacity.

Carbohydrate-processing enzymes depend on similar principles. They reduce complex carbohydrates into simpler sugars that can be transported across the intestinal membrane. When substrates are delivered in forms that match enzymatic requirements, breakdown proceeds efficiently. When delivery is irregular or when substrate load exceeds capacity, incomplete processing occurs, and a portion of these carbohydrates remains in the lumen.

Supplemental enzymes provide additional catalytic capacity within this framework. They increase the rate at which substrates are reduced when endogenous enzyme output is insufficient or when intake exceeds current capacity. Their effect is most pronounced when upstream preparation is already functional, because they integrate into an existing process and accelerate it. When structural preparation is weak, their impact is limited because they are acting on substrates that are not accessible.

Timing determines how effectively enzymes can operate. They must be present when substrates enter the intestine and remain active for the duration of the processing window. Coordinated motility ensures that substrates remain in contact with enzymes long enough for breakdown to occur. When motility is too rapid, contact time is reduced, and processing remains incomplete. When it is too slow, partially processed material accumulates, altering the internal environment.

Digestive enzymes therefore act within a defined sequence where structure determines access and access determines breakdown. Their role is to complete the conversion of macromolecules into absorbable forms, not to compensate for failures in earlier phases. When the sequence is aligned, enzymes operate efficiently and continuously. When it is not, their activity reflects the limitations imposed by incomplete preparation and disrupted timing.

Chapter 26

From Fragility to Flexibility

Fragility in digestion reflects a system that can only operate within a narrow range of conditions. Small changes in input, timing, or state produce disproportionate effects because each phase of the sequence is operating near its limit. Acid output is inconsistent, enzyme release does not match substrate load, bile flow is poorly timed, and motility lacks coordination. The system compensates rather than processes. Flexibility emerges when these same components are aligned and capable of adjusting to variation without losing function. The difference is not the presence of digestion, but the range over which it can operate without breakdown.

The transition from fragility to flexibility begins with restoring consistency in early-phase signaling and neural regulation. When the system reliably enters a state that supports digestion, secretory output and motility patterns become predictable. This predictability allows each phase to operate with sufficient capacity relative to incoming substrates. Variability in input no longer immediately disrupts the sequence because the system has margin. It can adjust without collapsing into incomplete processing.

Structural preparation is the next layer that expands flexibility. When gastric acid consistently unfolds proteins and alters the physical state of the meal, downstream processes receive substrates that are easier to handle. Bile organizes lipids into dispersed structures that remain accessible across a range of conditions. These preparatory steps reduce resistance within the system, allowing enzymes and transporters to function effectively even as inputs vary. Flexibility increases because the system is not dependent on precise conditions to achieve adequate processing.

Timing and coordination determine how well this flexibility is expressed. When gastric emptying, enzyme release, and bile flow are synchronized, the system can handle variations in meal size and composition without losing alignment. Substrates are delivered in a pattern that matches processing capacity, and motility maintains contact between substrates and digestive components. When timing is consistent, the system adapts to changes in input by adjusting output rather than failing.

Lipid digestion contributes to flexibility by providing a sustained substrate flow that stabilizes energy availability and signaling. Properly processed fats extend the delivery of energy beyond rapid fluctuations, allowing the system to operate under a wider range of conditions without instability. This stabilizing effect supports both metabolic and digestive flexibility, reducing the sensitivity of the system to short-term variation.

Microbial and immune responses also shift as flexibility increases. When digestion is complete and substrates are absorbed efficiently, less material reaches distal regions in a partially processed state. This reduces fermentation and lowers the variability of compounds generated within the intestine. The internal environment becomes more stable, and immune signaling reflects this stability. The system no longer reacts strongly to minor changes because the underlying conditions remain controlled.

Flexibility is expressed as tolerance to variation. Different foods, larger meals, or changes in timing no longer produce immediate disruption because the system can process them within its expanded capacity. This does not mean that all inputs are handled equally, but that the range of acceptable inputs has increased. The system adjusts its output to match the input rather than being overwhelmed by it.

Moving from fragility to flexibility therefore reflects the restoration and strengthening of the digestive sequence. Neural regulation establishes consistent activation, structural preparation reduces resistance, coordinated timing maintains alignment, and lipid processing stabilizes the system. As these elements integrate, the system gains the ability to operate across a wider range of conditions without losing function, and digestion becomes resilient rather than reactive.

Restored Resilience

Restored resilience reflects a digestive system that maintains function across changing conditions without losing sequence or efficiency. It is not defined by perfect inputs or rigid control. It is defined by the system's ability to absorb variation while continuing to process, transform, and deliver substrates in a stable manner. When resilience is present, digestion no longer depends on narrow conditions. The sequence holds under different meal sizes, compositions, and timing because each phase has sufficient capacity and coordination to adapt.

This stability begins with consistent neural regulation. The system reliably enters a state that supports digestion, allowing blood flow, secretion, and motility to align before and during intake. Because this activation is repeatable, the initial conditions of digestion no longer fluctuate widely from meal to meal. Gastric acid rises to levels that match protein load, pancreatic output aligns with incoming substrates, and bile flow responds proportionally to lipid presence. The sequence starts in the correct state rather than attempting to recover after the fact.

Structural preparation becomes dependable as a result. Proteins are consistently unfolded, lipids are dispersed into accessible forms, and the physical matrix of food is reduced in a way that supports downstream processing. This removes a major source of variability because enzymes and transport systems receive substrates that fall within their functional range. The system does not need to compensate for poorly prepared material, and efficiency remains high even as inputs change.

Coordination between phases reinforces this resilience. Gastric emptying aligns with intestinal capacity, preventing overload and maintaining a steady flow of substrates into the small intestine. Enzyme release and bile flow match this delivery, allowing breakdown to proceed without accumulation of partially processed material. Motility maintains contact time between substrates and digestive components, ensuring that each phase completes its function before progression. The sequence operates as a continuous chain rather than a series of disconnected steps.

Lipid processing provides a stabilizing influence that extends beyond the digestive tract. Properly emulsified and absorbed fats deliver substrates over an extended period, supporting steady energy availability and consistent signaling. This reduces the impact of short-term fluctuations in other substrates and contributes to overall system stability. When lipid digestion is reliable, it anchors the system, allowing other variations to be absorbed without disruption.

The internal environment of the intestine reflects this restored order. Reduced accumulation of incomplete substrates limits fermentation and stabilizes the chemical and physical conditions within the lumen. Microbial activity aligns with a consistent substrate supply rather than fluctuating loads, and immune signaling decreases as exposure to irregular or partially processed material declines. The system becomes quieter, not because it is inactive, but because it is operating without excess disturbance.

Resilience is ultimately expressed as the ability to maintain output under variation. Meals that differ in composition or size are processed without triggering downstream effects because the sequence remains intact. The system adjusts its activity to match input rather than being constrained by it. This reflects a return to a state where digestion operates according to its structure, with each phase supporting the next and the entire process maintaining stability across changing conditions.

Stable Digestion Across Conditions

Stable digestion across conditions reflects a system that maintains sequence, timing, and output despite variation in meal size, composition, and context. The defining feature is not uniform input but consistent processing. When the digestive sequence is intact, the system adjusts secretion, motility, and transport in proportion to what is consumed. Larger meals trigger greater acid production, increased enzyme release, and stronger bile flow. Smaller meals produce a scaled response. The relationship between input and output remains proportional, and the sequence holds without collapse.

This stability begins with reliable neural activation. The system consistently enters a state that supports digestion, allowing blood flow, secretion, and motility to align before intake. Because this activation is repeatable, the starting conditions for digestion do not fluctuate widely. Each meal begins with sufficient capacity already in place, and the system does not need to compensate for delayed or incomplete signaling. This reduces variability at the earliest stage and carries forward through the entire sequence.

Structural preparation remains consistent across different inputs. Gastric acid unfolds proteins and reduces the physical resistance of the meal regardless of its composition. Bile disperses lipids into accessible forms, allowing enzymatic activity to proceed without limitation. These preparatory steps ensure that downstream processes receive substrates that fall within their functional range. As a result, enzymes and transport systems operate under stable conditions even when the composition of the meal changes.

Coordination between phases maintains alignment as conditions vary. Gastric emptying adjusts to match the readiness of the small intestine, preventing overload and maintaining a controlled flow of substrates. Enzyme release and bile delivery scale with this flow, ensuring that breakdown keeps pace with input. Motility patterns adapt to maintain contact time between substrates and digestive components, allowing each phase to complete its function before progression. This coordination allows the system to handle variation without losing sequence.

Lipid processing contributes to stability by providing a sustained substrate flow that reduces reliance on rapidly fluctuating inputs. When fats are consistently emulsified and absorbed, they extend energy delivery over time and support steady signaling. This stabilizes both metabolic and digestive processes, allowing the system to absorb variation in other substrates without disruption.

The internal environment remains controlled when processing is complete. Reduced accumulation of partially processed material limits fermentation and stabilizes luminal conditions. Microbial activity reflects a steady substrate supply rather than fluctuating loads, and immune signaling remains proportional to actual conditions. This consistency reduces the likelihood that changes in input will produce exaggerated responses.

Stable digestion across conditions therefore reflects a system that has restored its sequence and expanded its capacity. Neural activation, structural preparation, coordinated timing, and efficient transport operate together to convert varying inputs into consistent outputs. The system no longer depends on narrow conditions to function. It adjusts to variation while maintaining alignment, allowing digestion to proceed with reliability across a range of circumstances.

Made in the USA
Monee, IL
05 November 2026

67914362R20128